Copyright © 2023 by Splash Publications

All rights reserved. No part of this book may be reproduced or used in any manner without written permission of the copyright owner except for the use of quotations in a book review.

First paperback edition June 2023

Book design by Splash Publications

ISBN: 9798397052061

SMOOTHIE RECIPES
5 INGREDIENTS OR LESS

TABLE OF CONTENTS

Introduction 1
Introduction 2
Disclaimer/Nutrition Symbols 3
Fruit Smoothies 4
- Strawberry Banana Bliss 5
- Mango Tango 5
- Peachy Keen 6
- Blueberry Blast 6
- Kiwi Delight 7
- Raspberry Refresher 7
- Watermelon Cooler 8
- Pineapple Paradise 8
- Green Apple Zing 9
- Mango Berry Medley 9
- Banana Peanut Butter Bliss 10
- Citrus Sunshine 10
- Mixed Berry Blast 11
- Tropical Delight 11
- Cherry Berry Burst 12
- Pearfectly Sweet 12
- Lemon Blueberry Refresher 13
- Raspberry Coconut Crush 13
- Melon Mint Madness 14
- Blackberry Banana Blitz 14

Green Smoothies 15
- Classic Green Goddess 16
- Kale Berry Blast 16
- Spinach Mango Tango 17
- Cucumber Melon Cooler 17
- Pineapple Spinach Splash 18
- Avocado Green Dream 18
- Minty Green Refresher 19
- Tropical Green Paradise 19
- Green Apple Spinach Splash 20
- Ginger Greens 20

Protein Smoothies 21
- Banana Berry Blast 22
- Chocolate Peanut Butter Power 22
- Vanilla Berry Protein 23
- Green Protein Boost 23
- Blueberry Almond Delight 24
- Tropical Mango Protein 24
- Chocolate Cherry Powerhouse 25
- Peanut Butter Banana Boost 25
- Coffee Protein Kick 26
- Raspberry Yogurt Protein 26

Protein Smoothies 27
- Peanut Butter Banana Boost 28
- Greek Yogurt Berry Blend 28

Green Power protein Shake 29
Blueberry Oat Powerhouse 29
Strawberry Cashew Cream 30
Pineapple Coconut Delight 30

Detox Smoothies 31
- Cucumber Lemon Detox 32
- Pineapple Kale Detox 32
- Blueberry Beet Detox 33
- Apple Cinnamon Detox 33
- Ginger Turmeric Detox 34
- Carrot Ginger Detox 34
- Avocado Detox 35
- Watermelon Mint Detox 35
- Berry Detox Blast 36
- Papaya Ginger Detox 36

Energy Smoothies 37
- Banana Berry Boost 38
- Green Powerhouse 38
- Mango Ginger Zing 39
- Pineapple Coconut Delight 39
- Citrus Energy Blast 40
- Chocolate Banana Power 40
- Berry Oat Burst 41
- Tropical Green Energizer 41
- Coffee Banana Kickstart 42
- Matcha Green Tea Boost 42

Seasonal Smoothies   43
- Summer Sunshine 44
- Fall Harvest 44
- Winter Wonderland 45
- Spring Green 45
- Spring Blossom 46
- Autumn Spice 46

3 Ingredient Smoothies 47
- Banana Berry Blast 48
- Mango Tango 48
- Pineapple Paradise 49
- Green Goodness 49
- Creamy Avocado Delight 50
- Berry Beet Blend 50
- Coconut Pineapple Refresher 51
- Tropical Sunrise 51
- Peanut Butter Bliss 52
- Strawberry Kiwi Crush 52
- Watermelon Lime Splash 53
- Blueberry Delight 53
- Chocolate Banana Shake 54
- Raspberry Lemonade 54

Index 65

CATEGORY BENEFITS

Fruit Smoothies:
The primary benefit of fruit smoothies is their delicious taste combined with a wide range of essential vitamins, minerals, and antioxidants. They provide a refreshing and enjoyable way to meet your daily fruit intake, supporting overall health and well-being.

Green Smoothies:
The primary benefit of green smoothies lies in their potent nutrient content derived from leafy green vegetables. They are an excellent source of vitamins, minerals, and antioxidants, helping to boost your immune system, improve digestion, and promote overall vitality.

Protein Smoothies:
The primary benefit of protein smoothies is their ability to support muscle growth, repair, and recovery. By including protein-rich ingredients like Greek yogurt, nut butter, or plant-based protein sources, these smoothies provide a convenient and delicious way to meet your protein needs and aid in maintaining a healthy body composition.

Detox Smoothies:
The primary benefit of detox smoothies is their ability to support the body's natural detoxification processes. These smoothies often include ingredients like leafy greens, citrus fruits, and detoxifying herbs, which help to eliminate toxins, support liver function, and promote overall cleansing and rejuvenation.

Energy Smoothies:
The primary benefit of energy smoothies is their ability to provide a natural and sustained energy boost. Packed with energizing ingredients like fruits, vegetables, healthy fats, and natural sweeteners, these smoothies provide a quick and wholesome source of fuel, enhancing mental and physical performance throughout the day.

No matter which smoothie category you choose, rest assured that they are all healthy and offer a plethora of benefits. Whether you opt for fruit smoothies bursting with natural sweetness, nutrient-dense green smoothies, protein-packed creations, detoxifying blends, or energizing concoctions, each category brings its unique nutritional profile and advantages. The key lies in incorporating a variety of smoothie categories into your routine to enjoy a well-rounded intake of vitamins, minerals, antioxidants, and essential nutrients. So, feel free to explore and mix things up.

INTRODUCTION

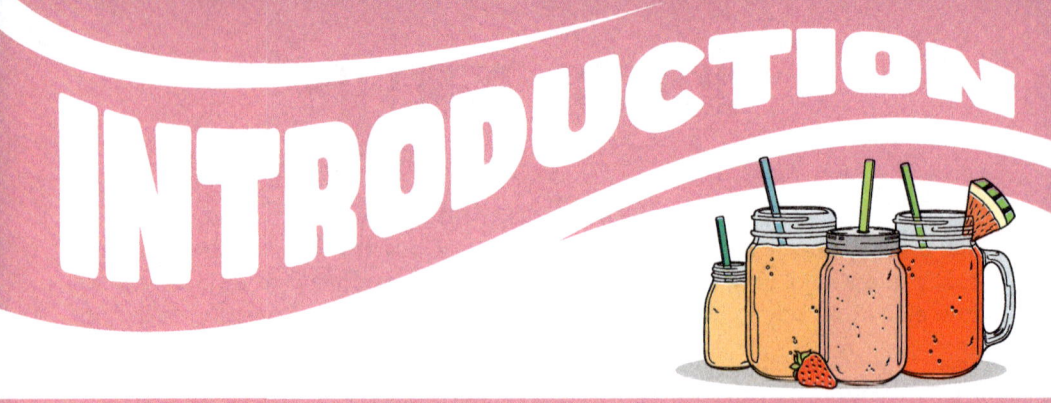

HERE'S THE LONG INTRODUCTION

Introducing 5 Ingredient or Less Smoothies – a delightful collection of recipes designed to bring ease and deliciousness into your smoothie-making adventures. In this book, we invite you to discover the beauty of simplicity as we unlock the secrets of creating nourishing and flavorful smoothies using just five ingredients or fewer.

Are you tired of complicated recipes with never-ending lists of ingredients? Do you yearn for a simpler approach that doesn't compromise on taste or nutrition? Look no further! "Simplicity in a Glass" is here to inspire and empower you to whip up a variety of mouthwatering smoothies without any fuss.

With our carefully curated selection of recipes, we aim to make your smoothie journey enjoyable and accessible to everyone, whether you're a seasoned smoothie enthusiast or a novice in the kitchen. Say goodbye to overwhelming trips to the grocery store in search of elusive ingredients. Embrace the joy of simplicity and let your creativity shine as you explore the possibilities within each recipe.

Inside this book, you'll find a wide range of smoothie recipes meticulously crafted to include only the essential ingredients, ensuring that each sip is bursting with flavor and packed with nutrients. From refreshing fruit-based blends to creamy and indulgent creations, we've got you covered. Explore categories like fruit smoothies, green smoothies, protein-rich options, dairy-free alternatives, breakfast delights, and even seasonal treats that capture the essence of each time of year.

Each recipe includes a precise list of ingredients, ensuring you have everything you need at hand. We've also provided accurate nutritional information and serving sizes to help you make informed choices (cant believe you're actually reading this) that align with your dietary preferences and goals. Whether you're seeking a post-workout refuel, a quick breakfast on the go, a satisfying snack, or a delightful dessert, there's a smoothie waiting to tempt your taste buds and nourish your body.

But "Simplicity in a Glass" is more than just a collection of recipes. We're here to inspire you to embrace the simplicity mindset, encouraging you to focus on quality ingredients, thoughtful combinations, and the joy of savoring a perfectly blended concoction. We believe that simplicity doesn't mean sacrificing flavor or health benefits. In fact, it's the opposite – by simplifying, we allow the natural flavors and nutritional goodness of each ingredient to shine through.

So, are you ready to embark on a delicious journey of simplicity? Join us as we dive into the world of five-ingredient or less smoothies, where convenience meets flavor, and where you'll discover that sometimes, less truly is more. Get ready to blend, sip, and savor your way to a healthier, more vibrant you. Cheers to "Simplicity in a Glass: 5 Ingredient or Less Smoothies" – your guide to effortless and delightful smoothie creations!

but no one is gonna read that, so basically...

Easy, tasty, very nice.

INTRODUCTION

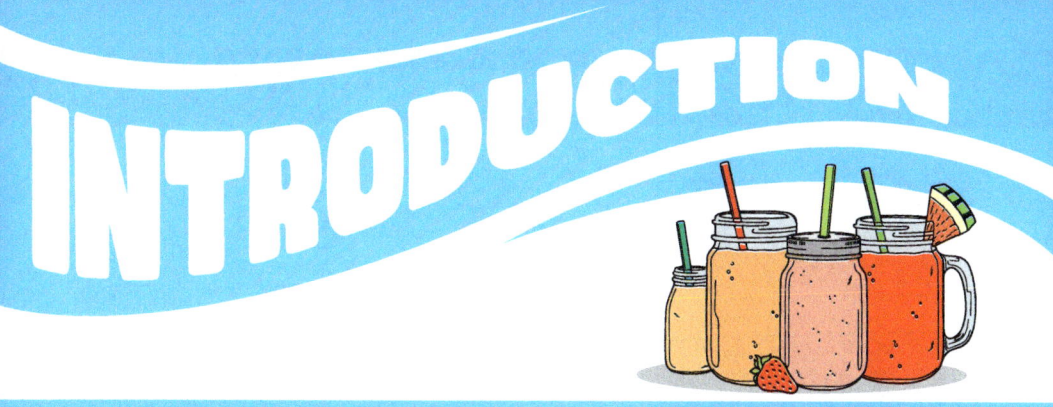

EQUIPMENT NEEDED

- Blender
- That's pretty much it
- Don't even need a blender if you can chop fast enough
- But a blender would be better
- Maybe a knife aswell
- And a small knife probably
- Find a big knife too, just in case
- Grater

BENEFITS OF SMOOTHIES

Contrary to popular belief smoothies do not give you super human abilities, so don't expect some blended fruit and vegetables to solve all your problems.

But it is a step closer to improving your health and well-being.

These delicious concoctions are packed with essential nutrients, including vitamins, minerals, and antioxidants, which support optimal bodily functions. They promote better digestion and gut health due to their high fiber content, helping to regulate bowel movements and prevent digestive issues. Additionally, these nutrient-dense beverages can aid in weight management by providing satiety and nourishment with lower calorie content.

Just remeber to have fun with it and the results will show eventually.

NUTRITION SYMBOLS

Calories   Protein   Total Fat   Carbohydrates   Fiber

Please note that the nutrition facts are per serving and may vary slightly depending on the specific brands and ingredients used plus the portion sizes. Additionally, these are only estimates and should be used as a general guide.

DISCLAIMER

The information provided in this smoothie recipe book is for general informational purposes only. While we have made every effort to ensure the accuracy and completeness of the content, we cannot guarantee the effectiveness or safety of the recipes and suggestions provided.

It is important to note that individuals may have different dietary needs, health conditions, or allergies that could impact their ability to consume certain ingredients or follow specific recipes. We strongly recommend consulting with a healthcare professional or registered dietitian before making any significant changes to your diet, particularly if you have specific health concerns or are on medication.

The recipes contained in this book are not intended to diagnose, treat, cure, or prevent any disease. The results and experiences obtained from consuming the smoothies may vary from person to person.

Readers should exercise caution and use their own discretion when preparing and consuming the smoothies. It is essential to carefully read the ingredient lists, nutritional information, and follow proper food safety guidelines, including storage, handling, and preparation techniques.

The authors, publishers, and contributors of this book cannot be held responsible for any adverse effects, allergic reactions, or damages that may arise from the use of the recipes or information provided. It is the responsibility of the reader to assess their individual needs, preferences, and health conditions before incorporating any smoothie recipe or ingredient into their diet.

By using this book, you acknowledge and agree to assume all risks associated with the preparation and consumption of the smoothies and waive any claims against the authors, publishers, and contributors.

FRUIT SMOOTHIES

In the following pages you will find
a bunch of fruit smoothie recipes.
You're welcome.

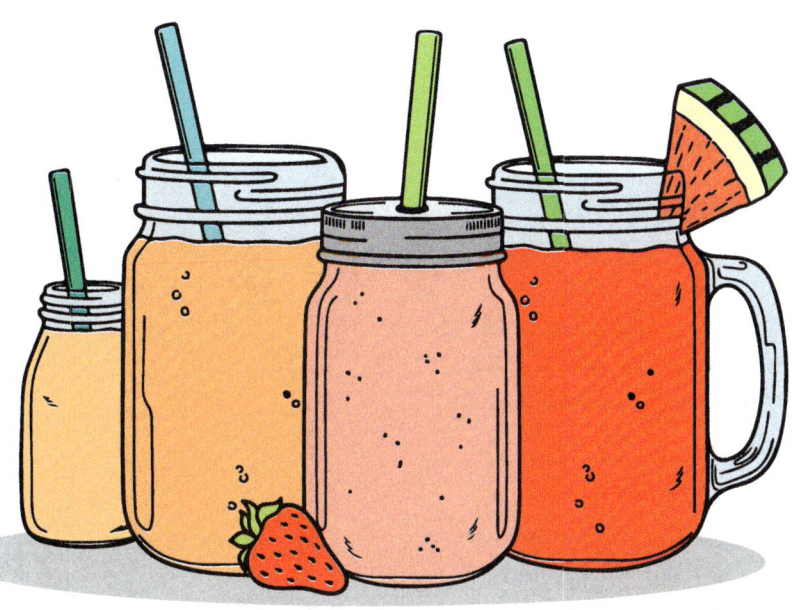

STRAWBERRY BANANA BLISS

180kcal
5g
1g
40g
4g

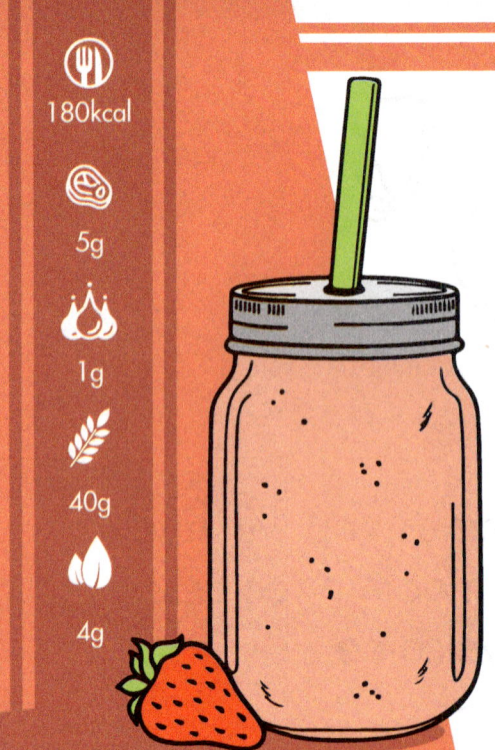

Ingredients:

- 1 cup strawberries
- 1 ripe banana
- 1/2 cup plain yogurt
- 1/2 cup orange juice
- 1 tablespoon honey (optional)

Add all the ingredients to the blender and blend untill the desired texture and consistency is reached

MANGO TANGO

Ingredients:

- 1 ripe mango
- 1/2 cup pineapple chunks
- 1/2 cup coconut milk
- 1/2 cup orange juice
- 1/2 cup ice cubes

Add all the ingredients to the blender and blend untill the desired texture and consistency is reached

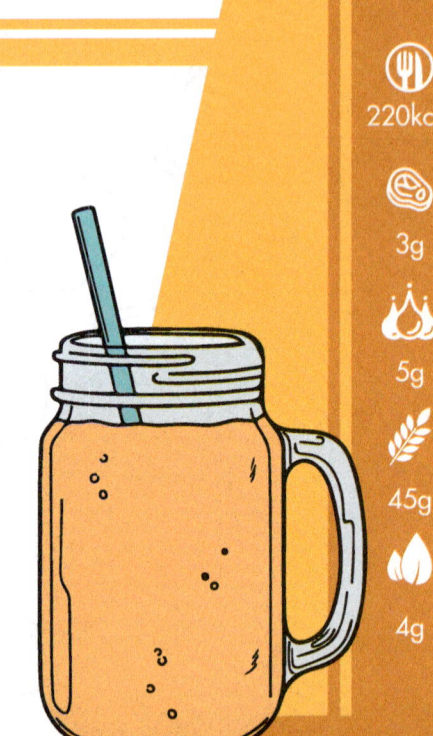

220kcal
3g
5g
45g
4g

PEACHY KEEN

Ingredients:

- 2 ripe peaches
- 1/2 cup almond milk
- 1/2 cup plain Greek yogurt
- 1/2 teaspoon vanilla extract
- 1/2 cup ice cubes

Add all the ingredients to the blender and blend untill the desired texture and consistency is reached

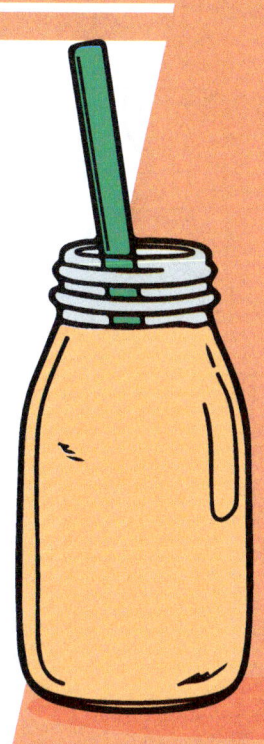

 150kcal

 7g

 3g

 28g

 3g

BLUEBERRY BLAST

Ingredients:

- 1 cup blueberries
- 1 ripe banana
- 1/2 cup almond milk
- 1/2 cup plain yogurt
- 1 tablespoon honey (optional)

Add all the ingredients to the blender and blend untill the desired texture and consistency is reached

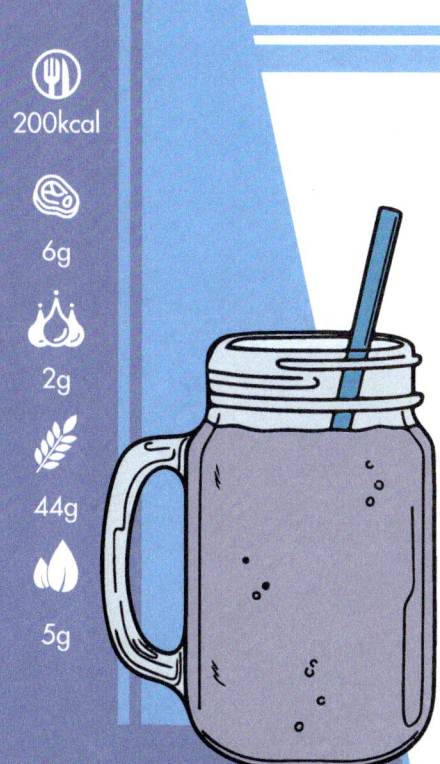

200kcal

6g

2g

44g

5g

KIWI DELIGHT

130kcal

3g

1g

30g

5g

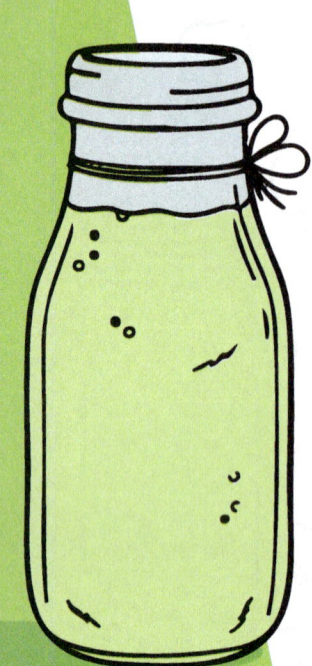

Ingredients:

- 2 ripe kiwis
- 1/2 cup pineapple chunks
- 1/2 cup coconut water
- 1/2 cup ice cubes

Add all the ingredients to the blender and blend untill the desired texture and consistency is reached

---

RASPBERRY REFRESHER

Ingredients:

- 1 cup raspberries
- 1/2 cup orange juice
- 1/2 cup coconut water
- 1/2 cup plain yogurt
- 1 tablespoon agave syrup (optional)

Add all the ingredients to the blender and blend untill the desired texture and consistency is reached

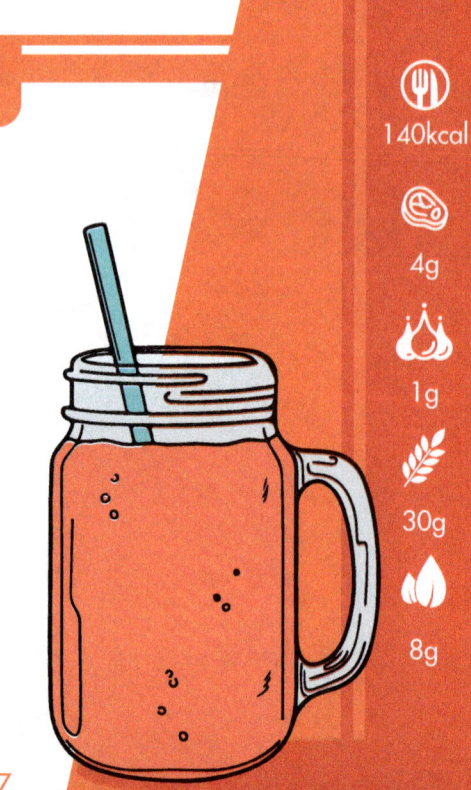

140kcal

4g

1g

30g

8g

WATERMELON COOLER

Ingredients:

- 2 cups diced water-melon
- 1/2 cup coconut water
- 1/2 cup lime juice
- 1 tablespoon mint leaves
- 1/2 cup ice cubes

Add all the ingredients to the blender and blend untill the desired texture and consistency is reached

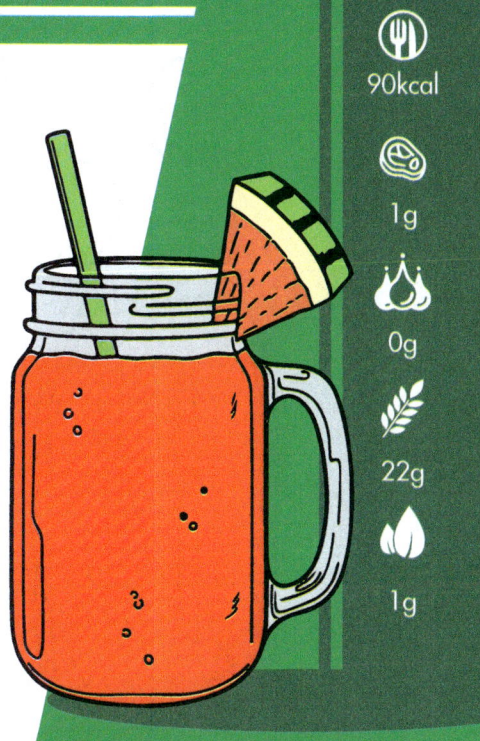

90kcal
1g
0g
22g
1g

180kcal

2g

4g

38g

3g

PINEAPPLE PARADISE

Ingredients:

- 1 cup pineapple chunks
- 1 ripe banana
- 1/2 cup coconut milk
- 1/2 cup orange juice
- 1/2 cup ice cubes

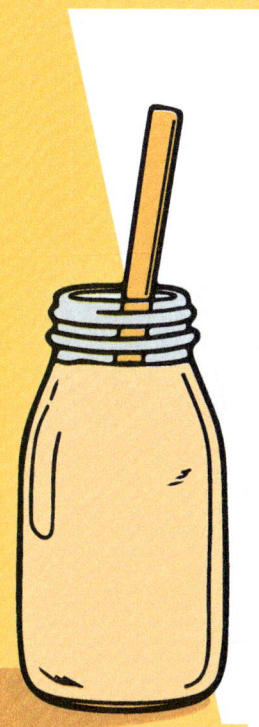

Add all the ingredients to the blender and blend untill the desired texture and consistency is reached

GREEN APPLE ZING

160kcal

5g

3g

30g

5g

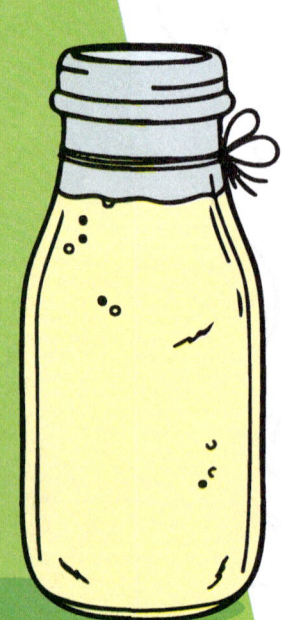

Ingredients:

- 2 green apples
- 1/2 cup almond milk
- 1/2 cup plain Greek yogurt
- 1/2 cup ice cubes

Add all the ingredients to the blender and blend untill the desired texture and consistency is reached

MANGO BERRY MEDLEY

Ingredients:

- 1 ripe mango
- 1/2 cup mixed berries (strawberries, blueberries, raspberries)
- 1/2 cup coconut water
- 1/2 cup plain yogurt
- 1 tablespoon honey

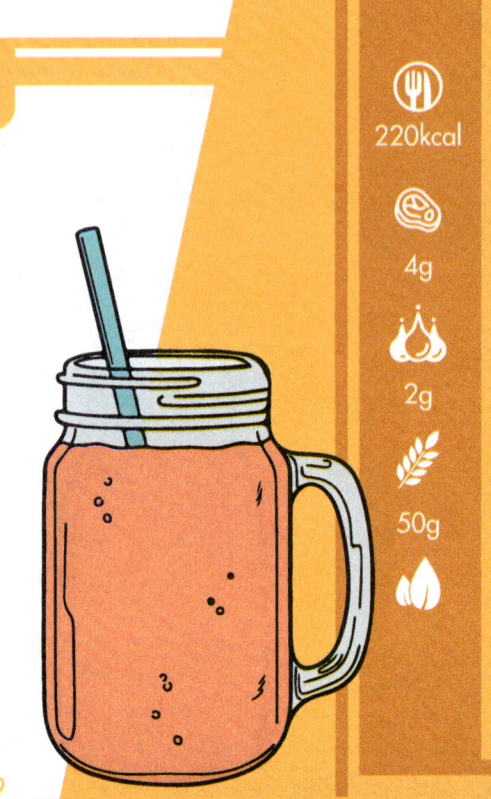

220kcal

4g

2g

50g

9

BANANA PEANUT BUTTER BLISS

Ingredients:

- 2 ripe bananas
- 2 tablespoons peanut butter
- 1 cup almond milk
- 1/2 teaspoon vanilla extract
- 1/2 cup ice cubes

Add all the ingredients to the blender and blend untill the desired texture and consistency is reached

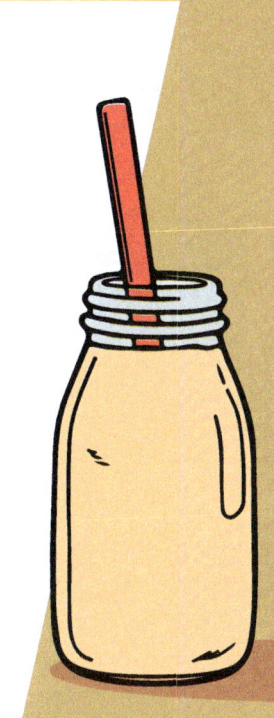

 320kcal

 8g

 14g

 45g

 6g

CITRUS SUNSHINE

Ingredients:

- 1 orange (or juice)
- 1/2 grapefruit
- 1/2 cup pineapple chunks
- 1/2 cup coconut water
- 1/2 cup ice cubes

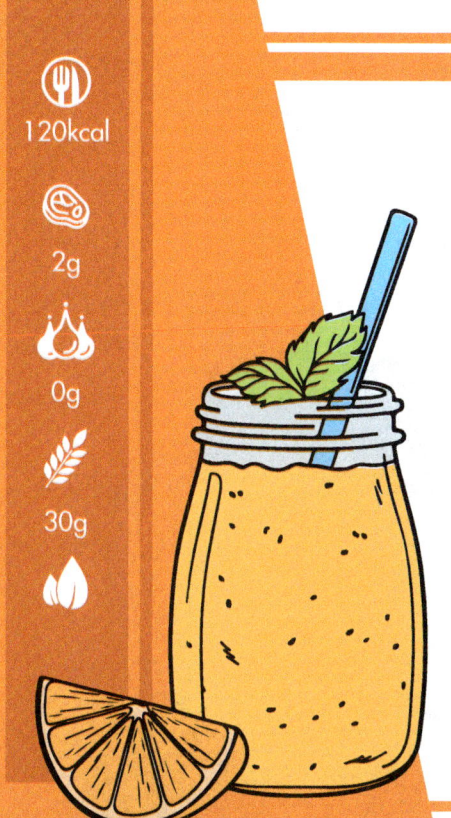

120kcal

2g

0g

30g

10

MIXED BERRY BLAST

160kcal
5g
2g
35g
6g

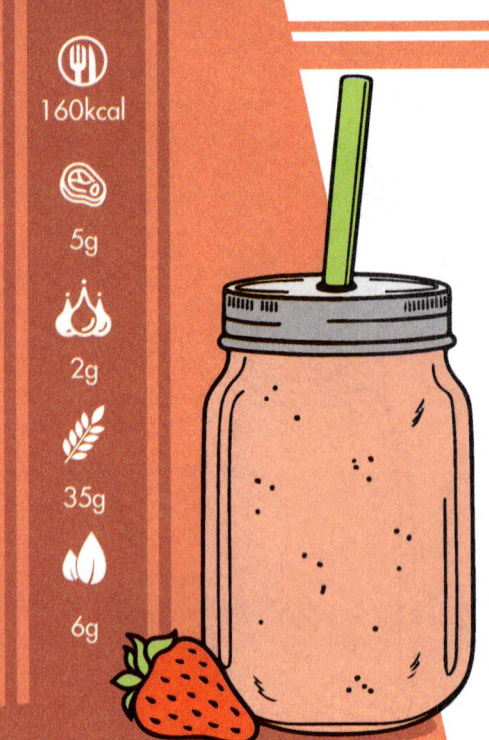

Ingredients:

- 1 cup mixed berries (strawberries, blueberries, raspberries)
- 1/2 cup almond milk
- 1/2 cup plain yogurt
- 1 tablespoon honey (optional)
- 1/2 cup ice cubes

Add all the ingredients to the blender and blend untill the desired texture and consistency is reached

TROPICAL DELIGHT

Ingredients:

- 1/2 cup pineapple chunks
- 1/2 cup mango chunks
- 1/2 cup coconut milk
- 1/2 cup orange juice
- 1/2 cup ice cubes

Add all the ingredients to the blender and blend untill the desired texture and consistency is reached

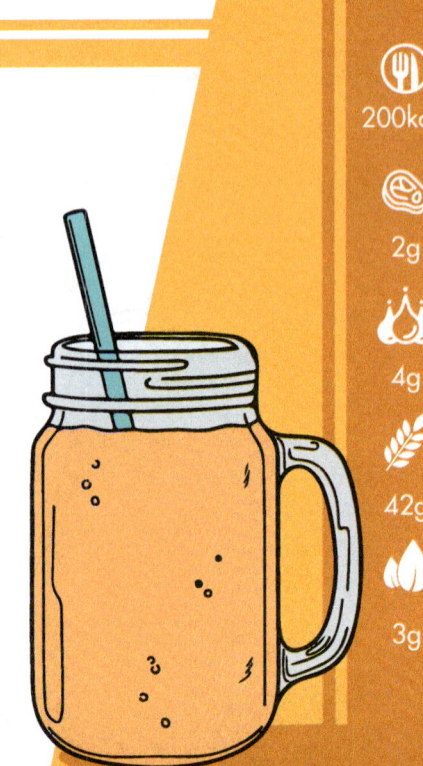

200kcal
2g
4g
42g
3g

CHERRY BERRY BURST

Ingredients:

- 1 cup cherries, pitted
- 1/2 cup mixed berries (strawberries, blueberries, raspberries)
- 1/2 cup almond milk
- 1/2 cup plain Greek yogurt
- 1/2 cup ice cubes

Add all the ingredients to the blender and blend untill the desired texture and consistency is reached

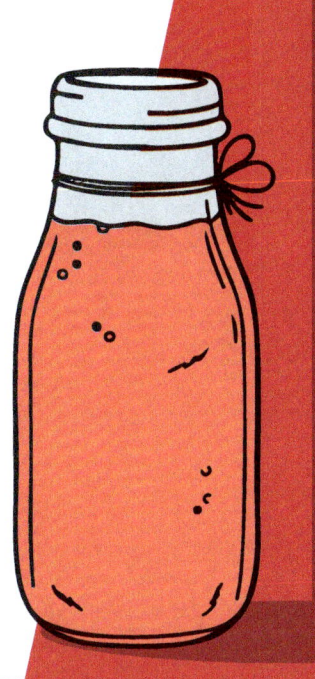

180kcal

6g

2g

35g

6g

150kcal

3g

2g

35g

6g

PEARFECTLY SWEET

Ingredients:

- 2 ripe pears
- 1/2 cup almond milk
- 1/2 teaspoon honey (optional)
- 1/2 cup ice cubes

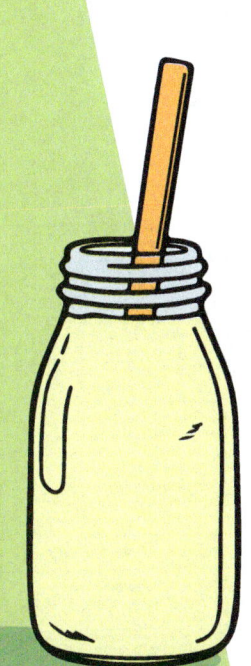

Add all the ingredients to the blender and blend untill the desired texture and consistency is reached

LEMON BLUEBERRY REFRESHER

140kcal

4g

2g

30g

5g

Ingredients:

- 1 cup blueberries
- Juice of 1 lemon
- 1/2 cup coconut water
- 1/2 cup plain yogurt
- 1/2 cup ice cubes

Add all the ingredients to the blender and blend untill the desired texture and consistency is reached

RASPBERRY COCONUT CRUSH

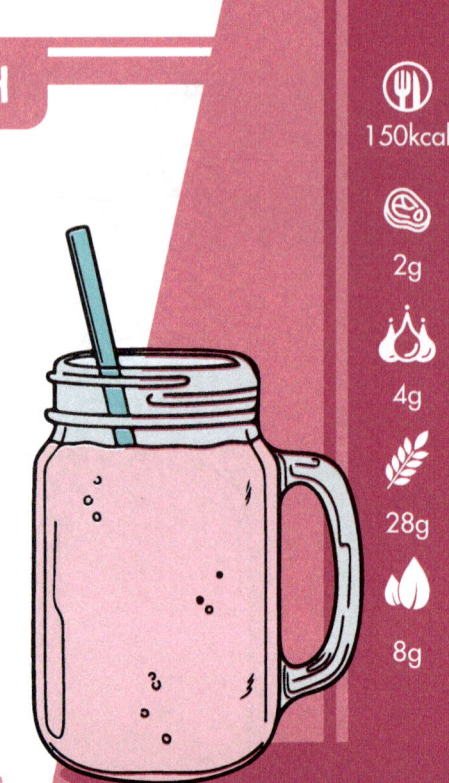

150kcal

2g

4g

28g

8g

Ingredients:

- 1 cup raspberries
- 1/2 cup coconut milk
- 1/2 cup orange juice
- 1 tablespoon agave syrup (optional)
- 1/2 cup ice cubes

Add all the ingredients to the blender and blend untill the desired texture and consistency is reached

MELON MINT MADNESS

Ingredients:

- 2 cups diced honey-dew melon
- 1/4 cup fresh mint leaves
- 1/2 cup coconut water
- Juice of 1 lime
- 1/2 cup ice cubes

Add all the ingredients to the blender and blend untill the desired texture and consistency is reached

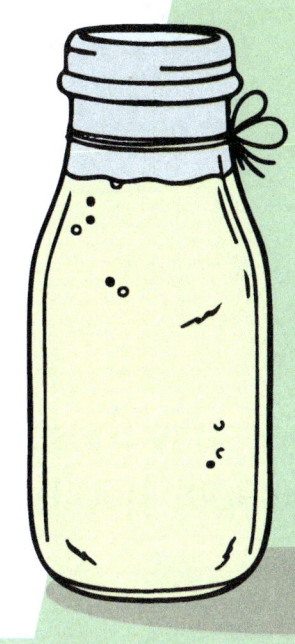

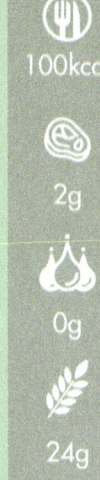
100kcal
2g
0g
24g
2g

BLACKBERRY BANANA BLITZ

Ingredients:

- 1 cup blackberries
- 1 ripe banana
- 1/2 cup almond milk
- 1/2 cup plain yogurt
- 1 tablespoon honey (optional)

Add all the ingredients to the blender and blend untill the desired texture and consistency is reached

180kcal

5g

2g

38g

8g

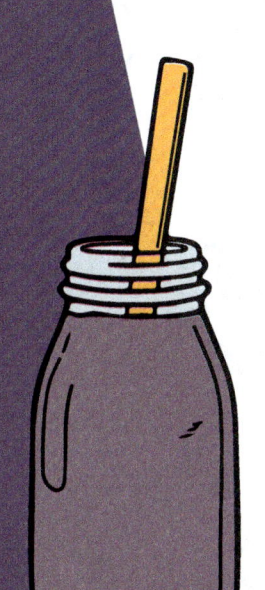

GREEN SMOOTHIES

Apparently these next smoothies are like super healthy for some reason.

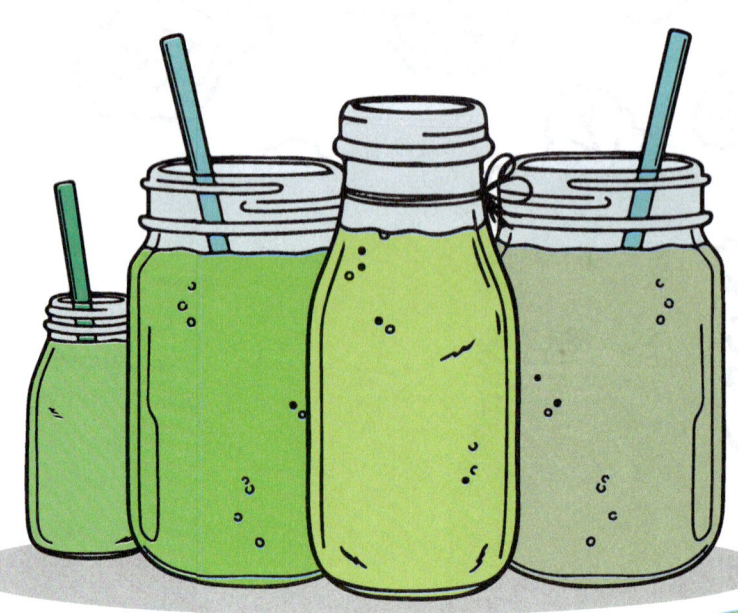

GREEN GODDESS

Ingredients:

- 2 cups spinach leaves
- 1 ripe banana
- 1/2 cup pineapple chunks
- 1/2 cup coconut water
- Juice of 1 lime

Add all the ingredients to the blender and blend untill the desired texture and consistency is reached

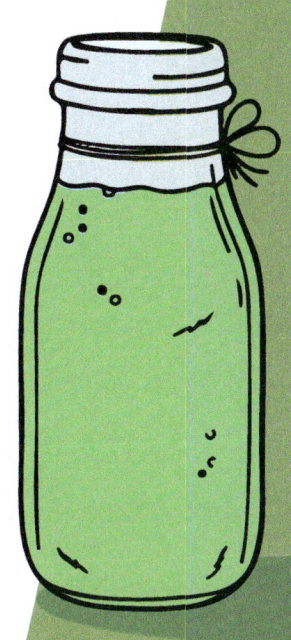

130kcal

3g

1g

33g

5g

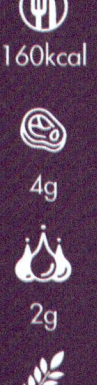
160kcal

4g

2g

36g

7g

KALE BERRY BLAST

Ingredients:

- 2 cups kale leaves
- 1 cup mixed berries (strawberries, blueberries, raspberries)
- 1/2 cup almond milk
- 1 tablespoon honey (optional)
- 1/2 cup ice cubes

Add all the ingredients to the blender and blend untill the desired texture and consistency is reached

160kcal
4g
1g
39g
5g

SPINACH MANGO TANGO

Ingredients:

- 2 cups spinach leaves
- 1 ripe mango
- 1/2 cup orange juice
- 1/2 cup coconut water
- 1/2 cup ice cubes

Add all the ingredients to the blender and blend untill the desired texture and consistency is reached

CUCUMBER MELON COOLER

Ingredients:

- 1 cup diced cucumber
- 2 cups diced honey-dew melon
- 1/2 cup coconut water
- Juice of 1 lime
- 1/2 cup ice cubes

Add all the ingredients to the blender and blend untill the desired texture and consistency is reached

90kcal
2g
0g
22g
2g

PINEAPPLE SPINACH SPLASH

Ingredients:

- 2 cups spinach leaves
- 1 cup pineapple chunks
- 1/2 cup coconut milk
- 1/2 cup orange juice
- 1/2 cup ice cubes

Add all the ingredients to the blender and blend untill the desired texture and consistency is reached

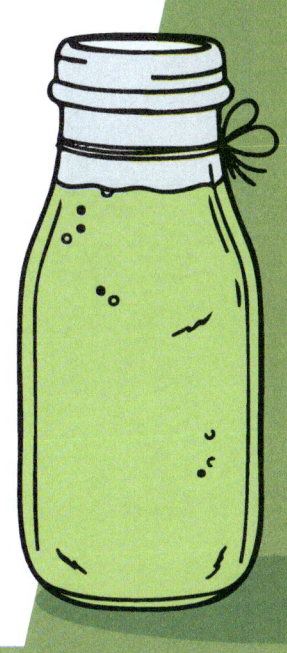

140kcal

3g

4g

30g

4g

AVOCADO GREEN DREAM

Ingredients:

- 1 ripe avocado
- 2 cups spinach leaves
- 1/2 cup almond milk
- Juice of 1 lime
- 1 tablespoon honey (optional)

Add all the ingredients to the blender and blend untill the desired texture and consistency is reached

240kcal

5g

17g

21g

12g

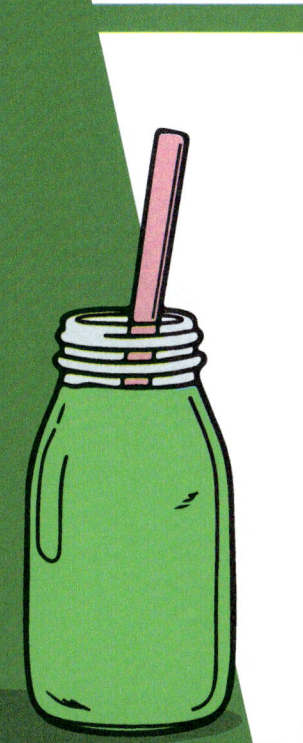

MINTY GREEN REFRESHER

100kcal
3g
1g
26g
5g

Ingredients:

- 2 cups spinach leaves
- 1/2 cup fresh mint leaves
- 1/2 cup coconut water
- 1/2 cup pineapple chunks
- 1/2 cup ice cubes

Add all the ingredients to the blender and blend untill the desired texture and consistency is reached

TROPICAL GREEN PARADISE

Ingredients:

- 2 cups spinach leaves
- 1/2 cup pineapple chunks
- 1/2 cup mango chunks
- 1/2 cup coconut milk
- Juice of 1 lime

Add all the ingredients to the blender and blend untill the desired texture and consistency is reached

180kcal
4g
4g
36g
6g

19

GREEN APPLE SPINACH SPLASH

Ingredients:

- 2 cups spinach leaves
- 1 green apple
- 1/2 cup cucumber slices
- 1/2 cup coconut water
- Juice of 1 lemon

Add all the ingredients to the blender and blend untill the desired texture and consistency is reached

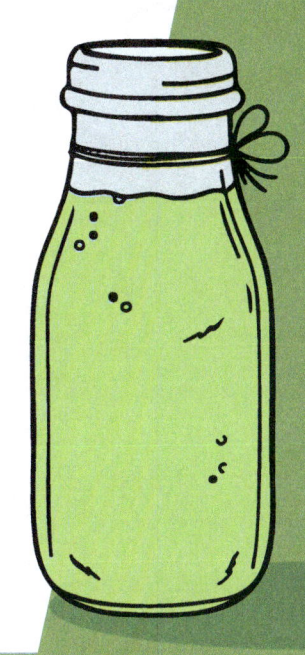

120kcal
3g
1g
28g
5g

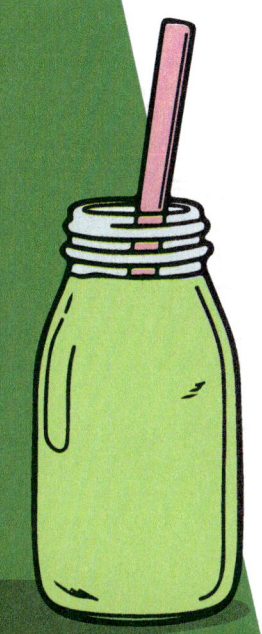

90kcal

3g

1g

22g

5g

GINGER GREENS

Ingredients:

- 2 cups spinach leaves
- 1/2 cup cucumber slices
- 1/2 cup pineapple chunks
- 1 teaspoon grated ginger
- 1/2 cup coconut water

Add all the ingredients to the blender and blend untill the desired texture and consistency is reached

PROTEIN SMOOTHIES

Make you strong.

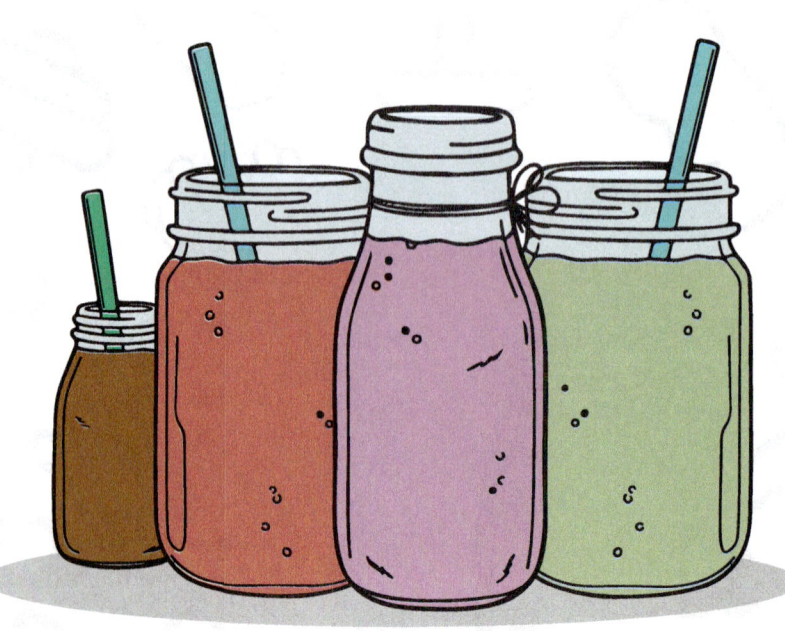

BANANA BERRY BLAST

Ingredients:

- 1 ripe banana
- 1 cup mixed berries (strawberries, blueberries, raspberries)
- 1 cup almond milk
- 1 scoop vanilla protein powder
- 1/2 cup ice cubes

Add all the ingredients to the blender and blend untill the desired texture and consistency is reached

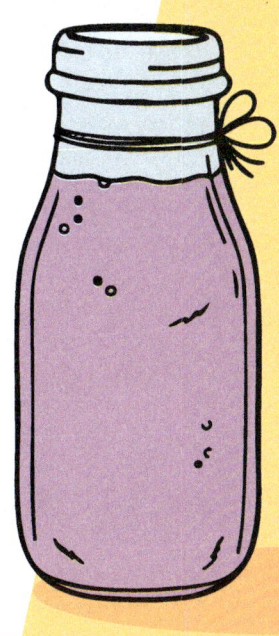

 280kcal

 25g

 4g

 40g

 8g

CHOCOLATE PEANUT BUTTER POWER

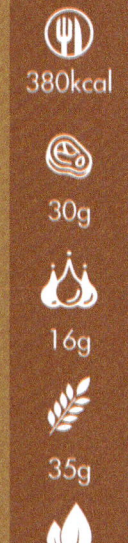

380kcal

30g

16g

35g

6g

Ingredients:

- 1 cup almond milk
- 1 scoop chocolate protein powder
- 2 tablespoons peanut butter
- 1 ripe banana
- 1/2 cup ice cubes

Add all the ingredients to the blender and blend untill the desired texture and consistency is reached

VANILLA BERRY

240kcal
25g
4g
30g
6g

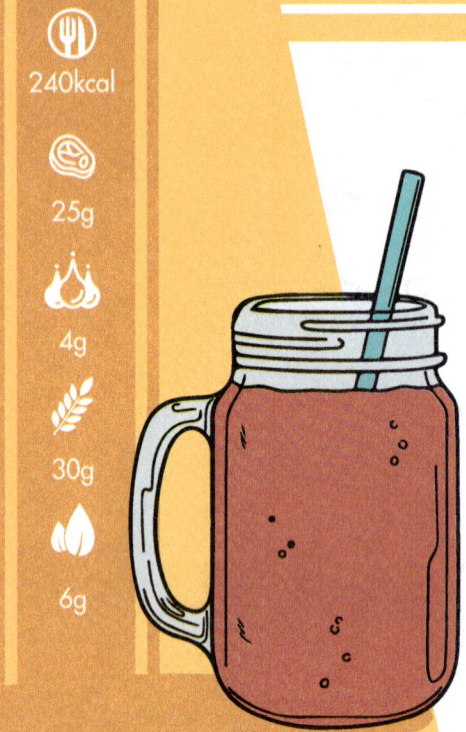

Ingredients:

- 1 cup mixed berries (strawberries, blueberries, raspberries)
- 1 cup almond milk
- 1 scoop vanilla protein powder
- 1 tablespoon honey (optional)
- 1/2 cup ice cubes

Add all the ingredients to the blender and blend untill the desired texture and consistency is reached

GREEN PROTEIN BOOST

260kcal
25g
4g
35g
6g

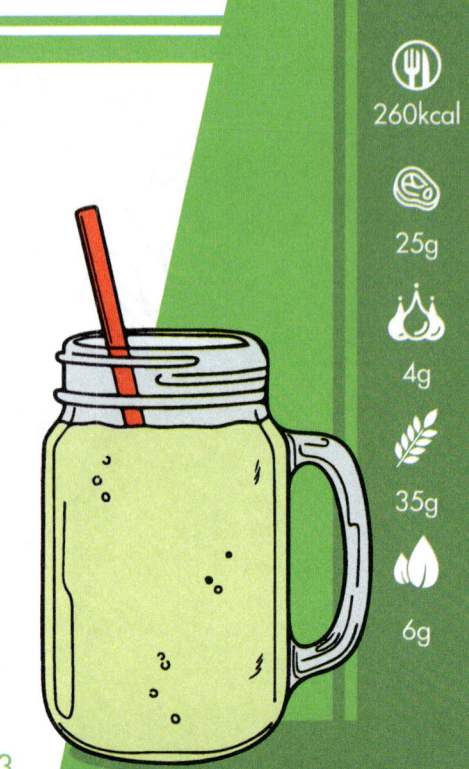

Ingredients:

- 2 cups spinach leaves
- 1 ripe banana
- 1 cup almond milk
- 1 scoop vanilla protein powder
- 1/2 cup ice cubes

Add all the ingredients to the blender and blend untill the desired texture and consistency is reached

BLUEBERRY ALMOND DELIGHT

Ingredients:

- 1 cup blueberries
- 1 cup almond milk
- 1 scoop vanilla protein powder
- 2 tablespoons almond butter
- 1/2 cup ice cubes

Add all the ingredients to the blender and blend untill the desired texture and consistency is reached

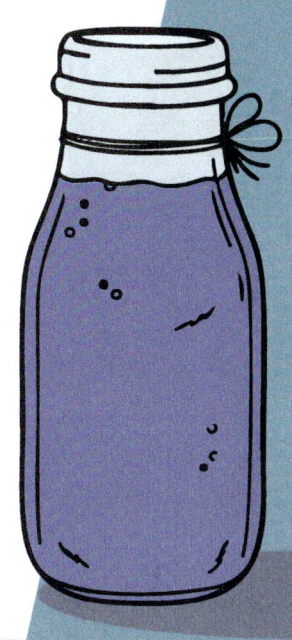

330kcal

25g

16g

30g

7g

TROPICAL MANGO PROTEIN

310kcal

25g

6g

45g

8g

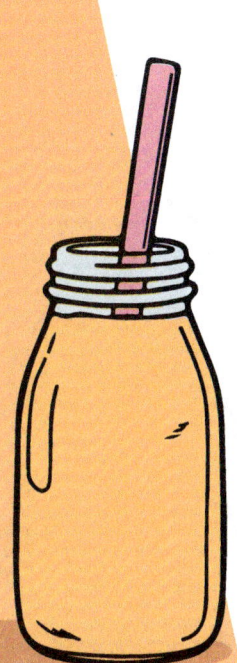

Ingredients:

- 1 ripe mango
- 1 cup coconut water
- 1 scoop vanilla protein powder
- 1 tablespoon chia seeds
- 1/2 cup ice cubes

Add all the ingredients to the blender and blend untill the desired texture and consistency is reached

CHOCOLATE CHERRY POWERHOUSE

320kcal
30g
8g
35g
8g

Ingredients:

- 1 cup cherries, pitted
- 1 cup almond milk
- 1 scoop chocolate protein powder
- 1 tablespoon cocoa powder
- 1/2 cup ice cubes

Add all the ingredients to the blender and blend untill the desired texture and consistency is reached

---

PEANUT BUTTER BANANA BOOST

Ingredients:

- 2 ripe bananas
- 1 cup almond milk
- 2 tablespoons peanut butter
- 1 scoop vanilla protein powder
- 1/2 cup ice cubes

Add all the ingredients to the blender and blend untill the desired texture and consistency is reached

410kcal
30g
14g
50g
7g

25

COFFEE PROTEIN KICK

Ingredients:

- 1 cup brewed coffee, chilled
- 1 cup almond milk
- 1 scoop chocolate protein powder
- 1 tablespoon almond butter
- 1/2 cup ice cubes

Add all the ingredients to the blender and blend untill the desired texture and consistency is reached

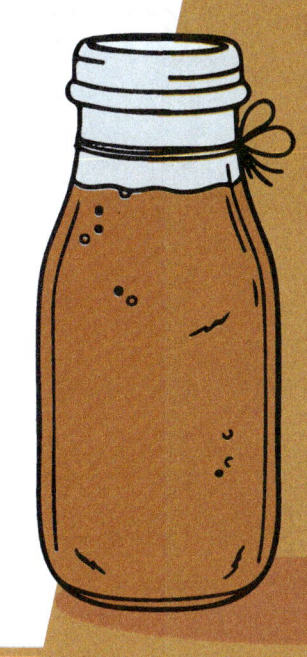

 220kcal

 25g

 10g

 15g

 4g

RASPBERRY YOGURT PROTEIN

Ingredients:

- 1 cup raspberries
- 1 cup plain Greek yogurt
- 1 scoop vanilla protein powder
- 1 tablespoon honey (optional)
- 1/2 cup ice cubes

Add all the ingredients to the blender and blend untill the desired texture and consistency is reached

 300kcal

 40g

 3g

 35g

 9g

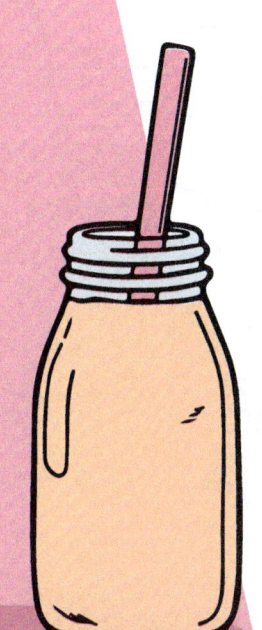

26

PROTEIN SMOOTHIES

Also make you strong,
but without protein powder.

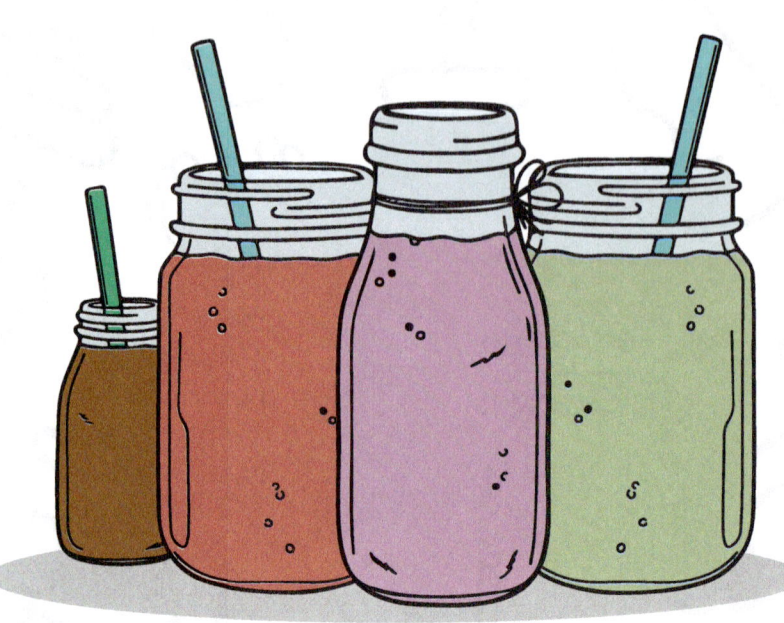

PEANUT BUTTER BANANA BOOST

Ingredients:

- 1 ripe banana
- 1 cup almond milk
- 2 tablespoons peanut butter
- 1 tablespoon chia seeds
- 1 tablespoon honey (optional)

Add all the ingredients to the blender and blend untill the desired texture and consistency is reached

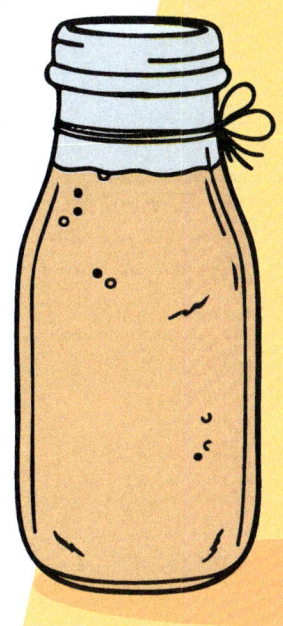

340kcal

9g

18g

40g

8g

GREEK YOGURT BERRY BLEND

220kcal

12g

5g

34g

9g

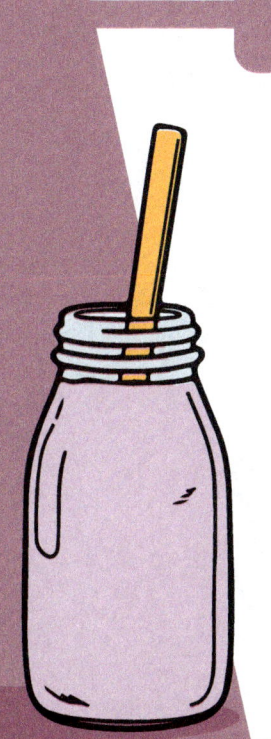

Ingredients:

- 1 cup mixed berries (strawberries, blueberries, raspberries)
- 1/2 cup Greek yogurt
- 1 cup almond milk
- 1 tablespoon honey (optional)
- 1 tablespoon flaxseeds

Add all the ingredients to the blender and blend untill the desired texture and consistency is reached

GREEN POWER PROTEIN SHAKE

250kcal

10g

4g

46g

7g

Ingredients:

- 2 cups fresh spinach
- 1 ripe banana
- 1/2 cup Greek yogurt
- 1 cup almond milk
- 1 tablespoon honey (optional)

Add all the ingredients to the blender and blend untill the desired texture and consistency is reached

BLUEBERRY OAT POWERHOUSE

Ingredients:

- 1 cup fresh or frozen blueberries
- 1/2 cup rolled oats
- 1 cup almond milk
- 1 tablespoon honey (optional)
- 1 tablespoon almond butter

Add all the ingredients to the blender and blend untill the desired texture and consistency is reached

300kcal

8g

9g

50g

9g

29

STRAWBERRY CASHEW CREAM

Ingredients:

- 1 cup fresh or frozen strawberries
- 1/2 cup cashews
- 1 cup almond milk
- 1 tablespoon honey (optional)
- 1/2 teaspoon vanilla extract

Add all the ingredients to the blender and blend untill the desired texture and consistency is reached

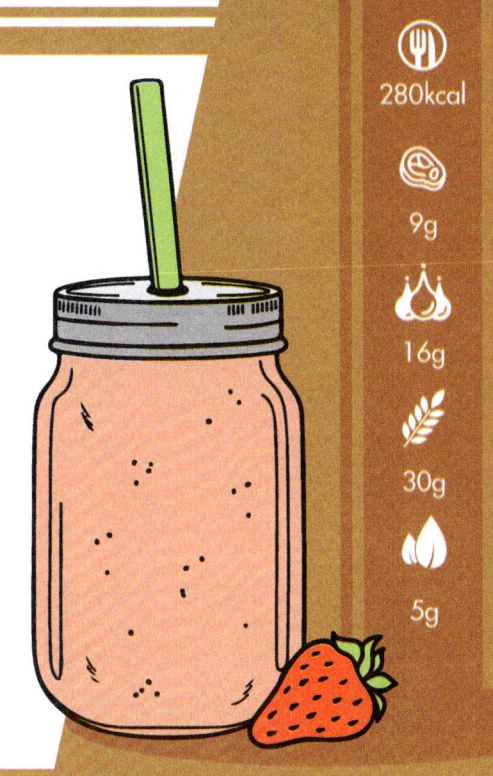

280kcal
9g
16g
30g
5g

PINEAPPLE COCONUT DELIGHT

Ingredients:

- 1 cup diced pineapple
- 1/2 cup coconut milk
- 1/2 cup Greek yogurt
- 1/2 cup orange juice
- 1 tablespoon shredded coconut

Add all the ingredients to the blender and blend untill the desired texture and consistency is reached

240kcal

9g

7g

36g

3g

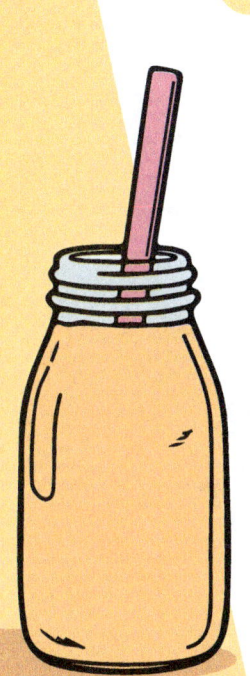

DETOX SMOOTHIES

I'm not even sure what these smoothies do.

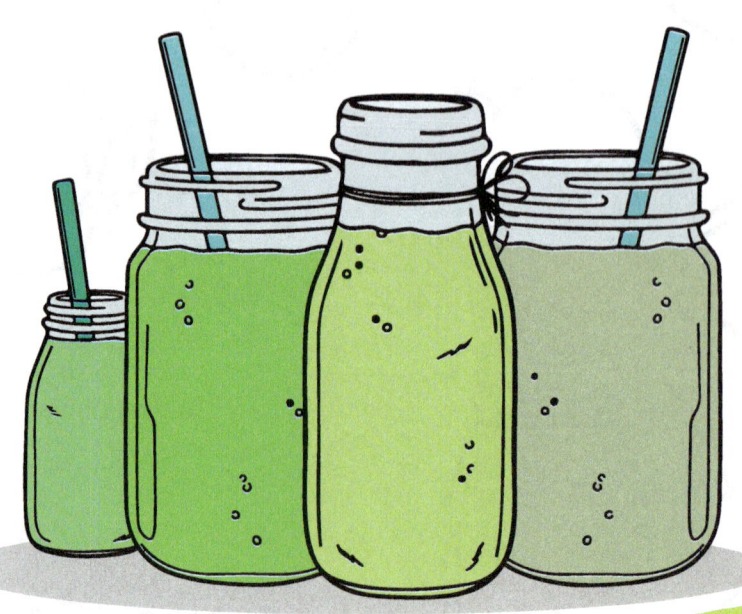

CUCUMBER LEMON DETOX

Ingredients:

- 1 cucumber
- 1 lemon
- 1 cup water
- 1 teaspoon grated ginger
- 1 handful of mint leaves

Add all the ingredients to the blender and blend untill the desired texture and consistency is reached

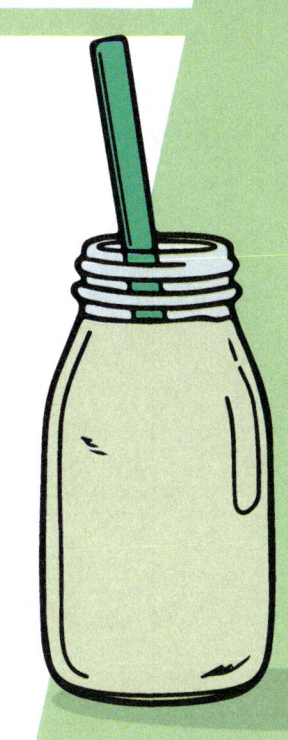

30kcal

1g

0g

8g

2g

PINEAPPLE KALE DETOX

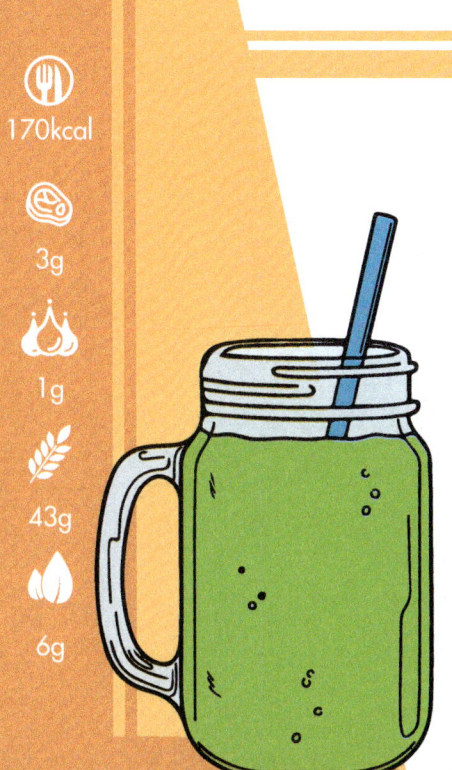

170kcal

3g

1g

43g

6g

Ingredients:

- 1 cup chopped kale
- 1 cup chopped pine-apple
- 1 banana
- 1/2 cup coconut water
- 1 teaspoon grated ginger

Add all the ingredients to the blender and blend untill the desired texture and consistency is reached

180kcal
4g
3g
40g
10g

BLUEBERRY BEET DETOX

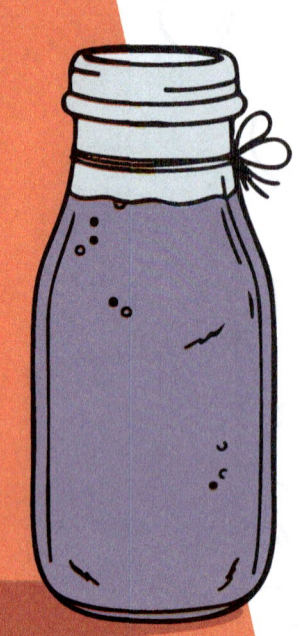

Ingredients:

- 1 cup blueberries
- 1 small beet
- 1 banana
- 1 cup water
- 1 tablespoon chia seeds

Add all the ingredients to the blender and blend untill the desired texture and consistency is reached

APPLE CINNAMON DETOX

Ingredients:

- 2 apples
- 1 cup water
- 1 teaspoon cinnamon
- 1/2 lemon
- 1 handful of spinach

Add all the ingredients to the blender and blend untill the desired texture and consistency is reached

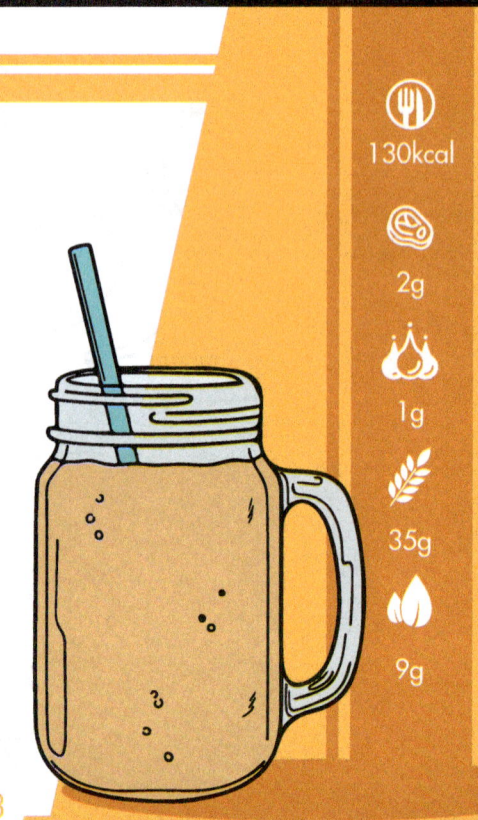

130kcal
2g
1g
35g
9g

33

GINGER TURMERIC DETOX

Ingredients:

- 1 banana
- 1 cup coconut water
- 1/2 teaspoon grated ginger
- 1/2 teaspoon ground turmeric
- 1/2 lemon

Add all the ingredients to the blender and blend untill the desired texture and consistency is reached

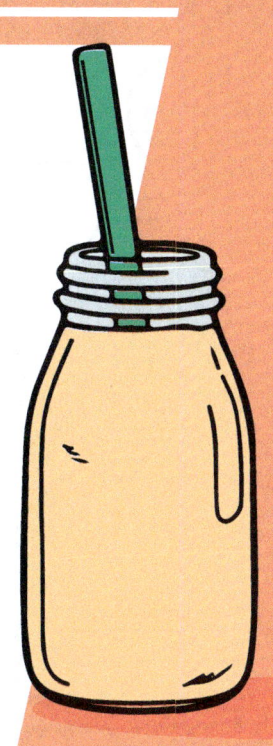

120kcal

2g

1g

30g

4g

CARROT GINGER DETOX

100kcal

3g

0g

26g

6g

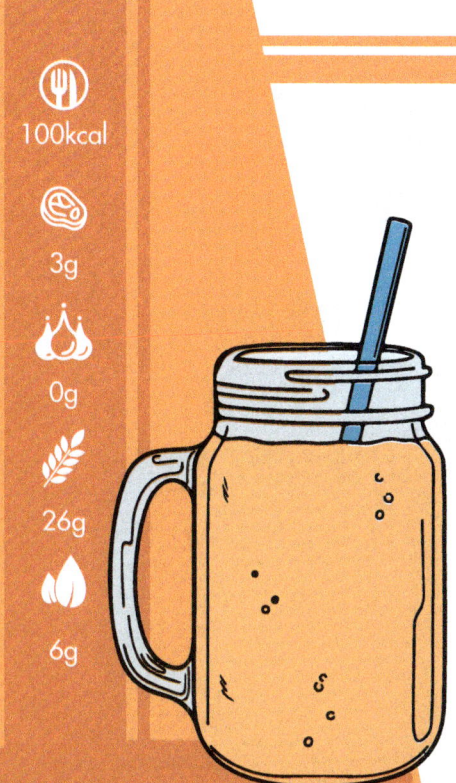

Ingredients:

- 2 large carrots
- 1 orange
- 1 inch fresh ginger
- 1 cup water
- 1 handful of spinach

Add all the ingredients to the blender and blend untill the desired texture and consistency is reached

AVOCADO DETOX

280kcal
5g
18g
30g
14g

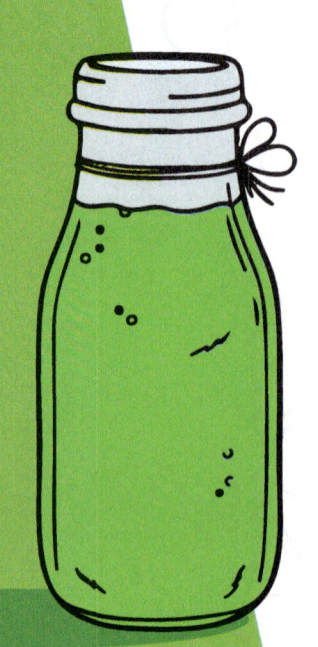

Ingredients:

- 1 ripe avocado
- 1 cup coconut water
- 1 lime
- 1 teaspoon honey
- 1 handful of spinach

Add all the ingredients to the blender and blend untill the desired texture and consistency is reached

BERRY DETOX BLAST

Ingredients:

- 1 cup mixed berries (strawberries, blueberries, raspberries)
- 1 cup coconut water
- 1 tablespoon chia seeds
- 1 tablespoon lemon juice
- 1 handful of spinach

Add all the ingredients to the blender and blend untill the desired texture and consistency is reached

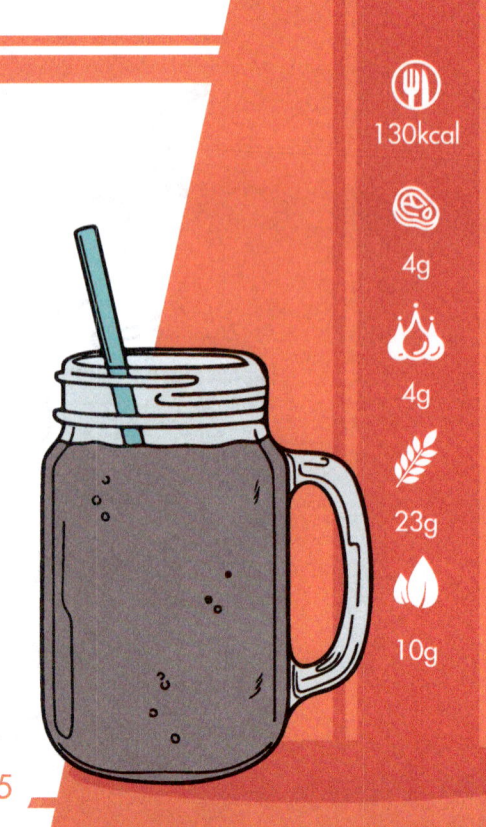

130kcal
4g
4g
23g
10g

WATERMELON MINT DETOX

Ingredients:

- 2 cups chopped watermelon
- 1/2 cup coconut water
- 1 handful of mint leaves
- 1/2 lemon
- 1 teaspoon honey

Add all the ingredients to the blender and blend untill the desired texture and consistency is reached

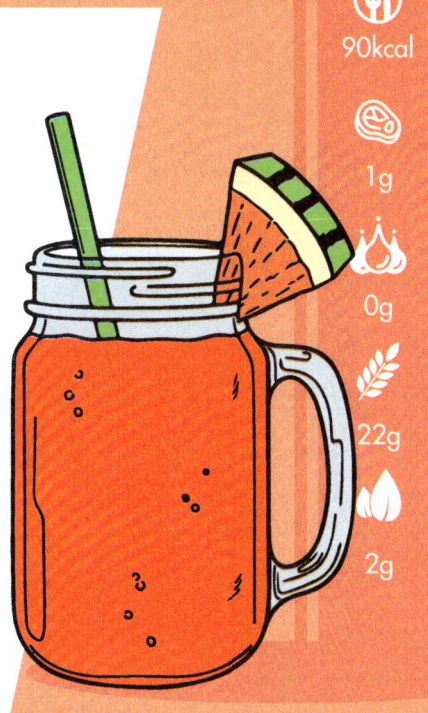

90kcal
1g
0g
22g
2g

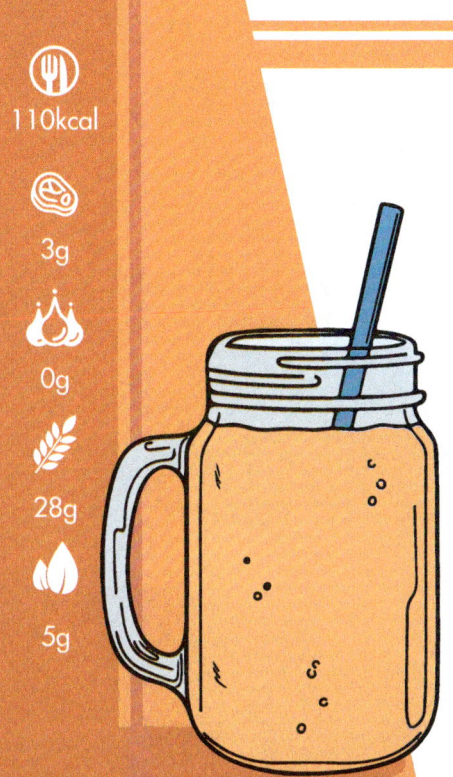

110kcal
3g
0g
28g
5g

PAPAYA GINGER DETOX

Ingredients:

- 1 cup diced papaya
- 1/2 cup coconut water
- 1/2 teaspoon grated ginger
- 1 tablespoon lime juice
- 1 handful of kale

Add all the ingredients to the blender and blend untill the desired texture and consistency is reached

ENERGY SMOOTHIES

You're only gonna need 1 hour of sleep a week with one of these smoothies.
(Not true, just in case someone tried it)

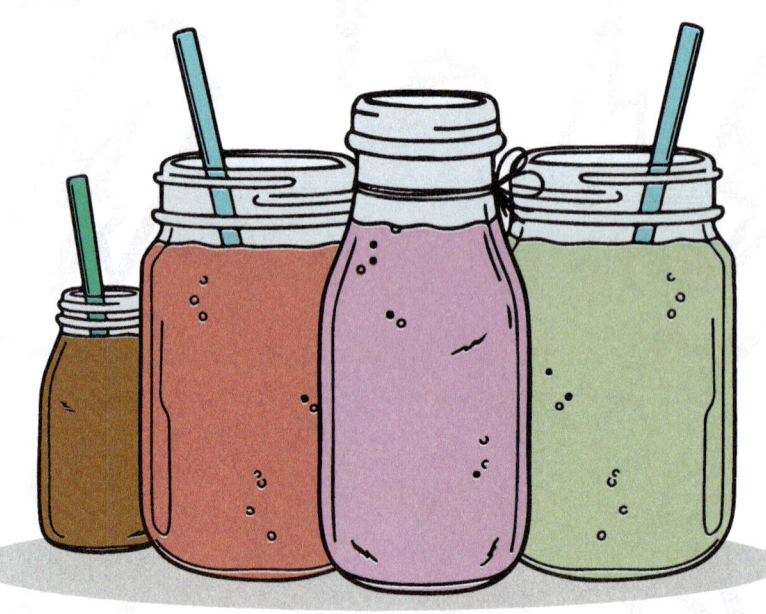

BANANA BERRY BOOST

Ingredients:

- 1 ripe banana
- 1 cup mixed berries (strawberries, blueberries, raspberries)
- 1 cup almond milk
- 1 tablespoon honey (optional)
- 1 tablespoon almond butter

Add all the ingredients to the blender and blend untill the desired texture and consistency is reached

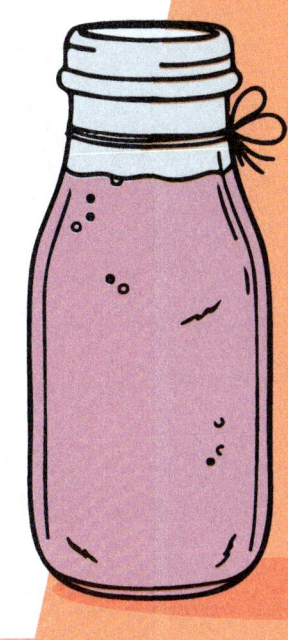

250kcal

4g

9g

41g

8g

GREEN POWERHOUSE

Ingredients:

- 2 cups spinach leaves
- 1 ripe banana
- 1 cup coconut water
- 1 tablespoon chia seeds
- 1/2 lemon

Add all the ingredients to the blender and blend untill the desired texture and consistency is reached

160kcal

5g

4g

29g

9g

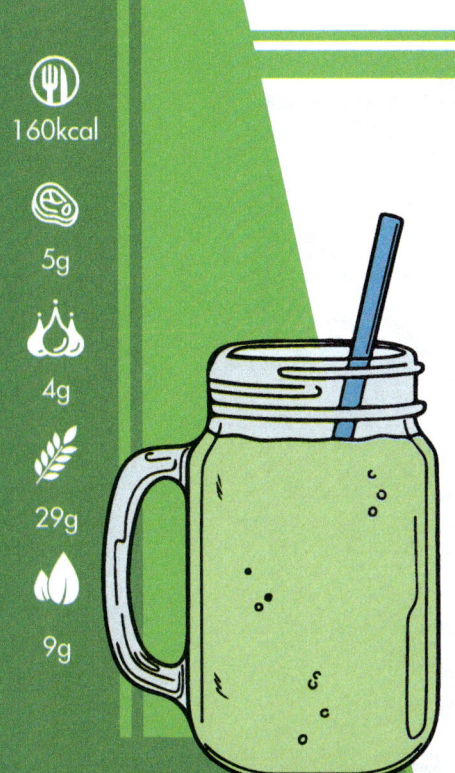

CHOCOLATE BANANA POWER

230kcal

6g

11g

32g

7g

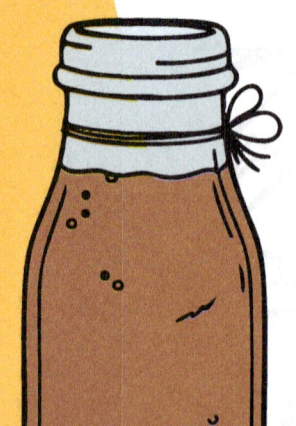

Ingredients:

- 1 ripe banana
- 1 cup almond milk
- 2 tablespoons cocoa powder
- 1 tablespoon almond butter
- 1 teaspoon honey (optional)

Add all the ingredients to the blender and blend untill the desired texture and consistency is reached

MANGO GINGER ZING

Ingredients:

- 1 cup chopped mango
- 1 inch fresh ginger
- 1 cup orange juice
- 1/2 cup almond milk
- 1 tablespoon honey (optional)

Add all the ingredients to the blender and blend untill the desired texture and consistency is reached

180kcal

2g

2g

42g

3g

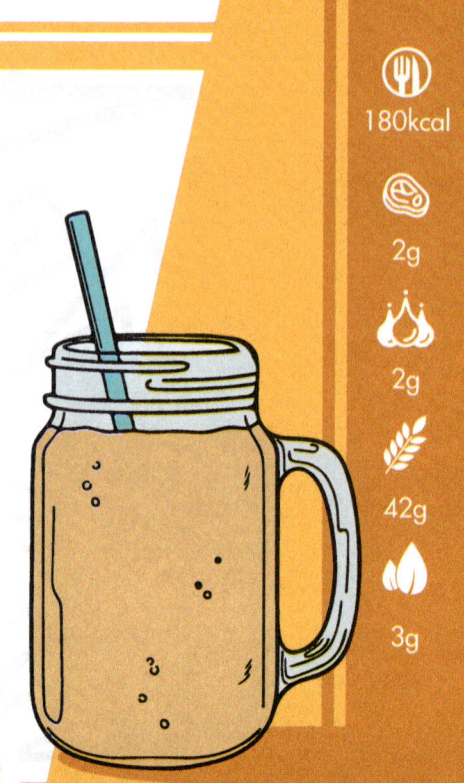

PINEAPPLE COCONUT DELIGHT

Ingredients:

- 1 cup chopped pine-apple
- 1/2 cup coconut milk
- 1/2 cup almond milk
- 1 tablespoon shredded coconut
- 1 teaspoon honey (optional)

Add all the ingredients to the blender and blend untill the desired texture and consistency is reached

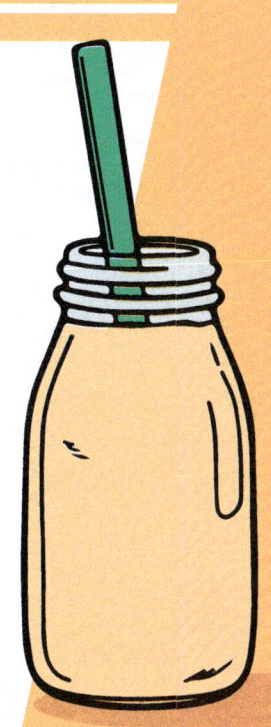

 180kcal

 2g

 10g

 24g

 3g

CITRUS ENERGY BLAST

Ingredients:

- 1 orange
- 1/2 grapefruit
- 1/2 lemon
- 1 cup coconut water
- 1 tablespoon honey (optional)

Add all the ingredients to the blender and blend untill the desired texture and consistency is reached

100kcal

1g

0g

26g

4g

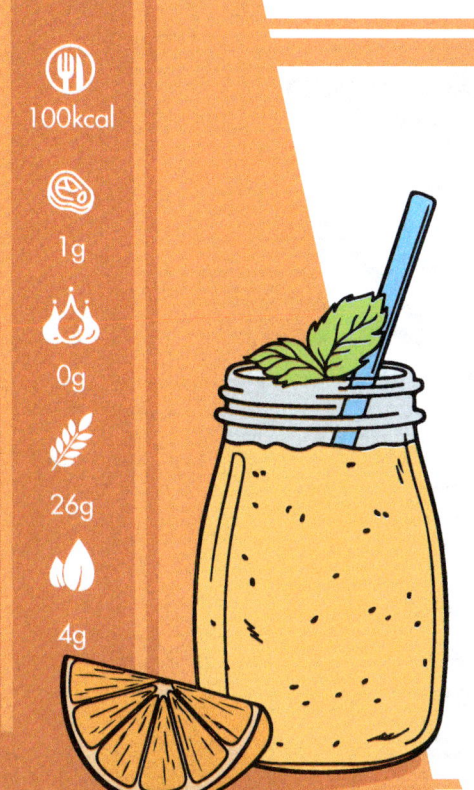

250kcal

6g

4g

50g

9g

BERRY OAT BURST

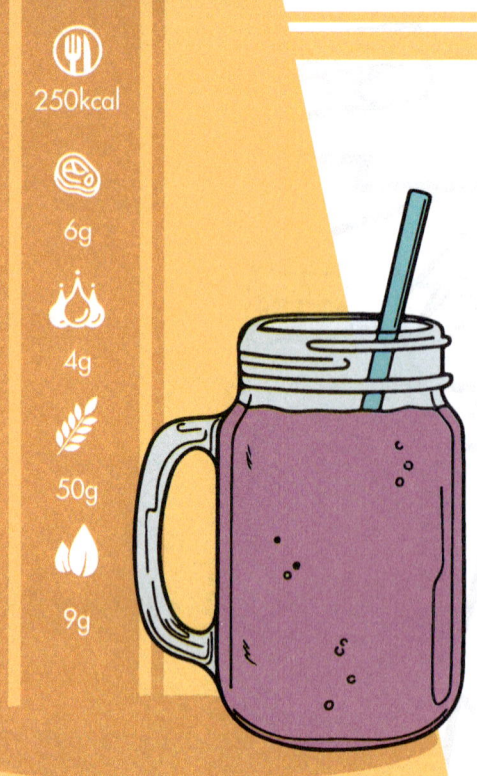

Ingredients:

- 1 cup mixed berries (strawberries, blueberries, raspberries)
- 1/2 cup rolled oats
- 1 cup almond milk
- 1 tablespoon honey (optional)
- 1/2 teaspoon vanilla extract

Add all the ingredients to the blender and blend untill the desired texture and consistency is reached

TROPICAL GREEN ENERGIZER

Ingredients:

- 1 cup chopped pineapple
- 1 ripe banana
- 1 cup spinach leaves
- 1 cup coconut water
- 1 tablespoon lime juice

Add all the ingredients to the blender and blend untill the desired texture and consistency is reached

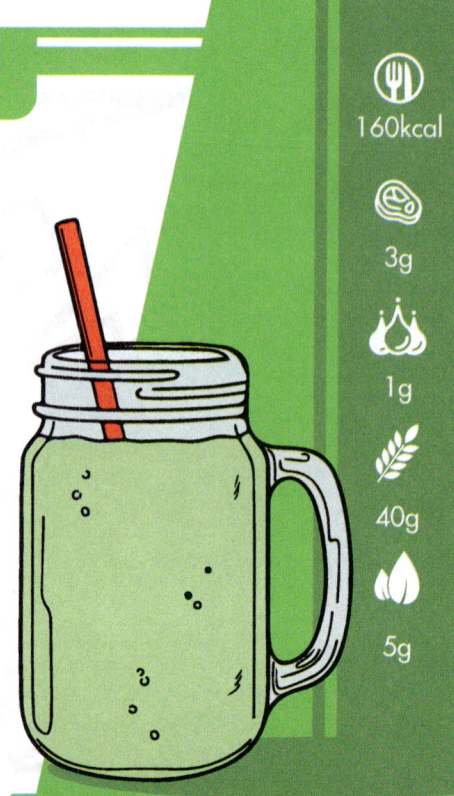

160kcal

3g

1g

40g

5g

41

MATCHA GREEN TEA BOOST

Ingredients:

- 1 teaspoon matcha green tea powder
- 1 cup almond milk
- 1 ripe banana
- 1 tablespoon honey (optional)
- 1/2 teaspoon vanilla extract

Add all the ingredients to the blender and blend untill the desired texture and consistency is reached

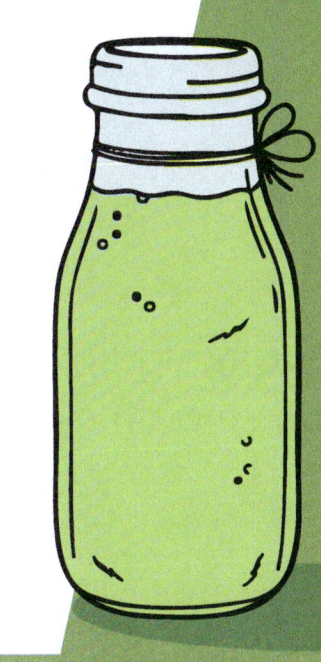

170kcal

3g

4g

32g

3g

160kcal

3g

7g

23g

4g

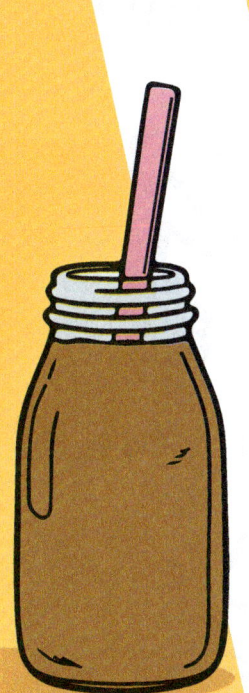

COFFEE BANANA KICKSTART

Ingredients:

- 1 ripe banana
- 1 cup brewed coffee, chilled
- 1/2 cup almond milk
- 1 tablespoon almond butter
- 1 teaspoon honey (optional)

Add all the ingredients to the blender and blend untill the desired texture and consistency is reached

SEASONAL SMOOTHIES

I'ts actually against the law to make any of these smoothies in the wrong season.

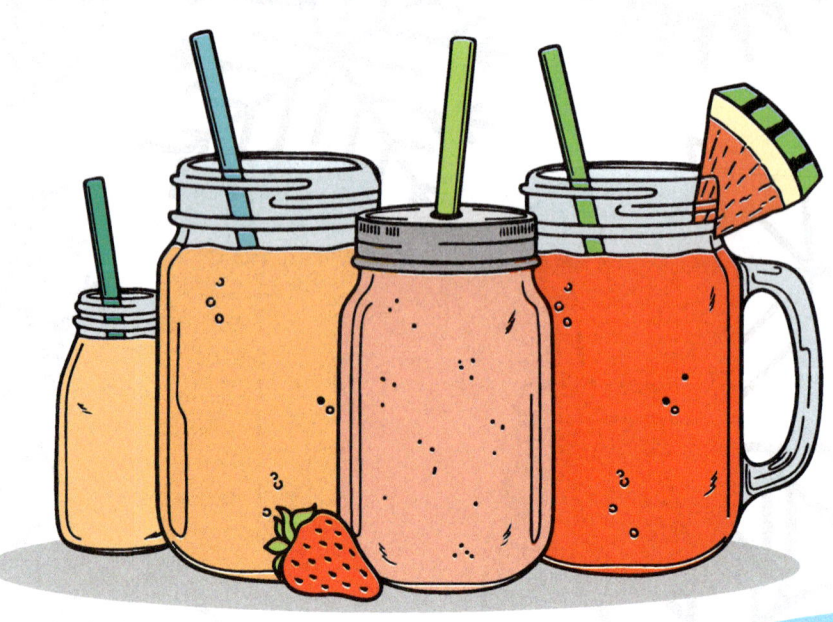

SUMMER SUNSHINE

Ingredients:

- 1 cup watermelon chunks
- 1/2 cup fresh pineapple
- 1/2 cup coconut water
- 1 tablespoon lime juice
- 1 tablespoon mint leaves

Add all the ingredients to the blender and blend untill the desired texture and consistency is reached

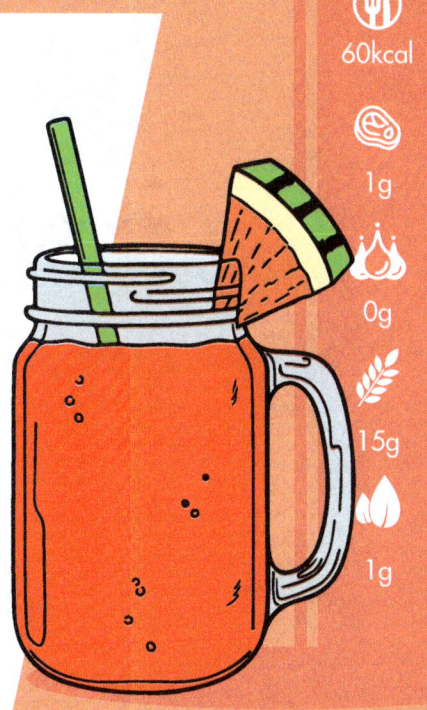

60kcal
1g
0g
15g
1g

FALL HARVEST

Ingredients:

- 1/2 cup cooked pumpkin
- 1 ripe banana
- 1 cup almond milk
- 1 tablespoon maple syrup
- 1/2 teaspoon pumpkin spice

Add all the ingredients to the blender and blend untill the desired texture and consistency is reached

120kcal
4g
3g
32g
5g

150kcal

9g

3g

25g

5g

WINTER WONDERLAND

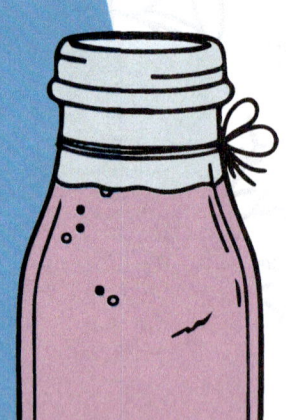

Ingredients:

- 1 cup mixed berries (cranberries, blueberries, raspberries)
- 1/2 cup Greek yogurt
- 1 cup almond milk
- 1 tablespoon honey (optional)
- 1/2 teaspoon vanilla extract

Add all the ingredients to the blender and blend untill the desired texture and consistency is reached

---

SPRING GREEN

Ingredients:

- 1 cup fresh spinach
- 1/2 cucumber
- 1 kiwi
- 1 cup coconut water
- 1 tablespoon lime juice

Add all the ingredients to the blender and blend untill the desired texture and consistency is reached

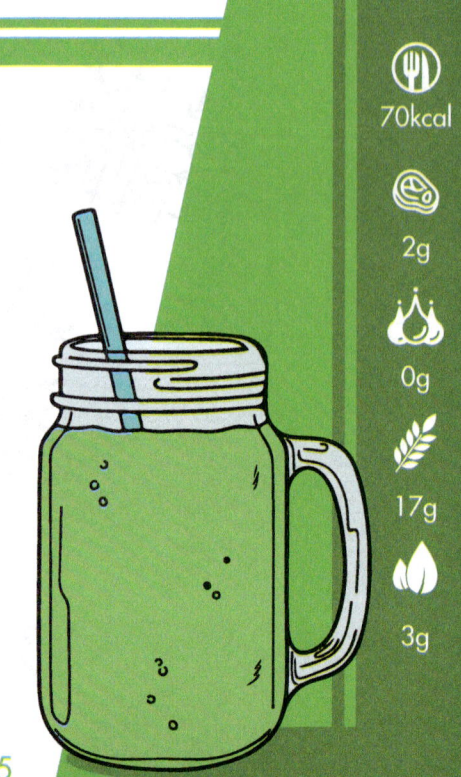

70kcal

2g

0g

17g

3g

45

SPRING BLOSSOM

Ingredients:

- 1 cup fresh strawberries
- 1 ripe banana
- 1 cup coconut water
- 1 tablespoon honey (optional)

Add all the ingredients to the blender and blend untill the desired texture and consistency is reached

130kcal
3g
1g
31g
5g

AUTUMN SPICE

120kcal
2g
3g
25g
6g

Ingredients:

- 1 ripe pear
- 1/2 cup unsweetened applesauce
- 1 cup almond milk
- 1/2 teaspoon cinnamon
- 1/4 teaspoon nutmeg

Add all the ingredients to the blender and blend untill the desired texture and consistency is reached

3 INGREDIENT SMOOTHIES

You can just use 1 ingredient if you really want to.

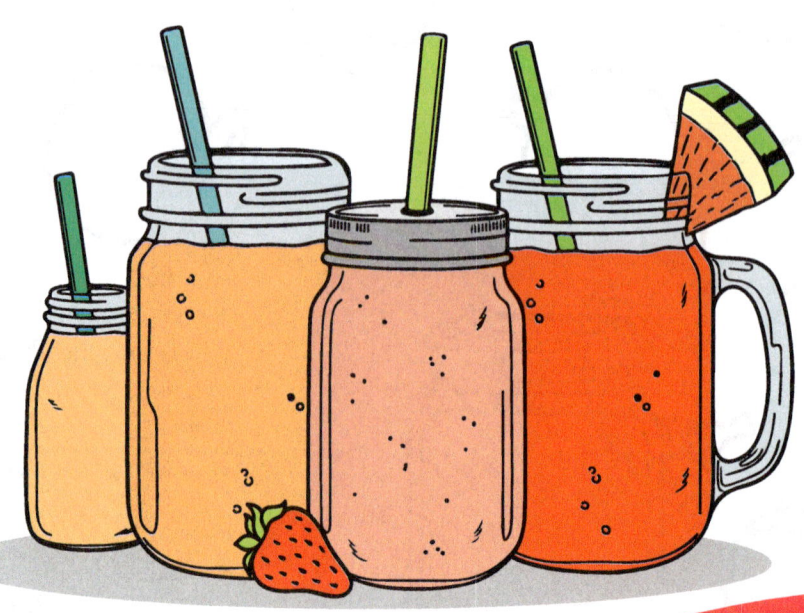

BANANA BERRY BLAST

Ingredients:

- 1 ripe banana
- 1 cup mixed berries (strawberries, blueberries, raspberries)
- 1/2 cup almond milk

Add all the ingredients to the blender and blend untill the desired texture and consistency is reached

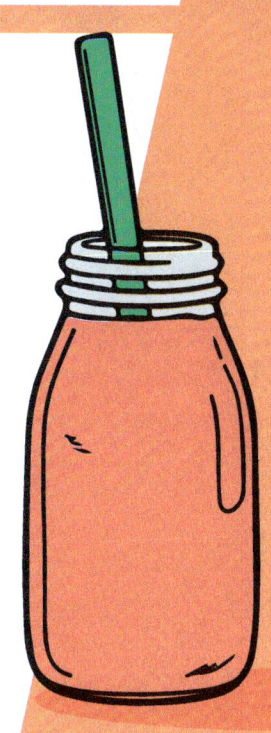

150kcal

2g

2g

35g

6g

MANGO TANGO

Ingredients:

- 1 ripe mango

- 1/2 cup Greek yogurt

- 1/2 cup orange juice

Add all the ingredients to the blender and blend untill the desired texture and consistency is reached

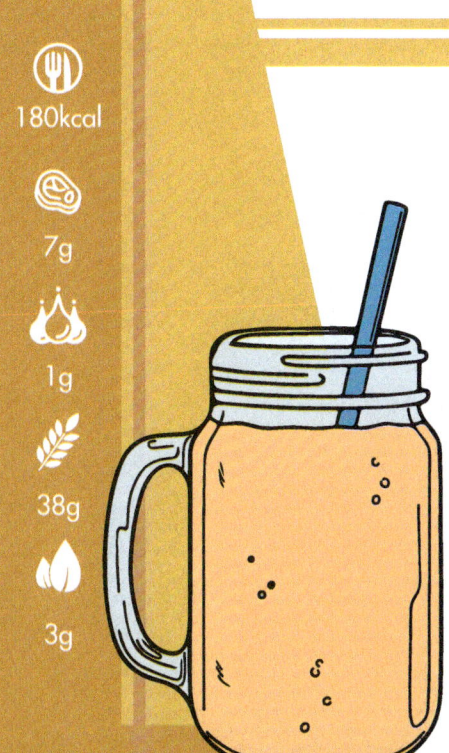
180kcal
7g
1g
38g
3g

GREEN GOODNESS

120kcal
3g
0g
29g
4g

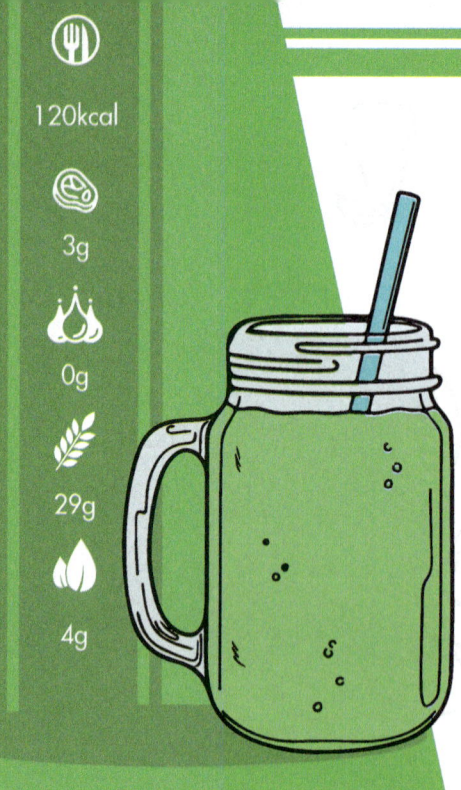

Ingredients:

- 2 cups spinach leaves
- 1 ripe banana
- 1/2 cup coconut water

Add all the ingredients to the blender and blend untill the desired texture and consistency is reached

PINEAPPLE PARADISE

Ingredients:

- 1 cup fresh pineapple chunks
- 1/2 cup coconut water
- Juice of 1 lime

Add all the ingredients to the blender and blend untill the desired texture and consistency is reached

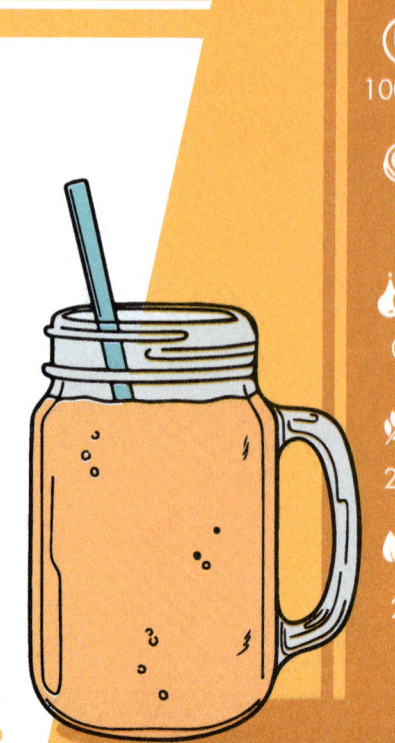

100kcal
1g
0g
25g
2g

49

CREAMY AVOCADO DELIGHT

Ingredients:

- 1 ripe avocado
- 1 cup almond milk
- 1 tablespoon honey (optional)

Add all the ingredients to the blender and blend untill the desired texture and consistency is reached

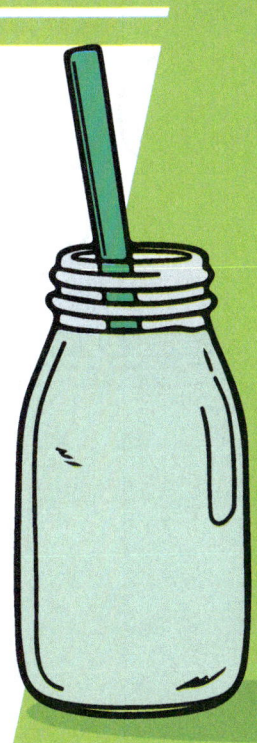

220kcal

3g

15g

22g

7g

BERRY BEET BLEND

140kcal

3g

1g

33g

8g

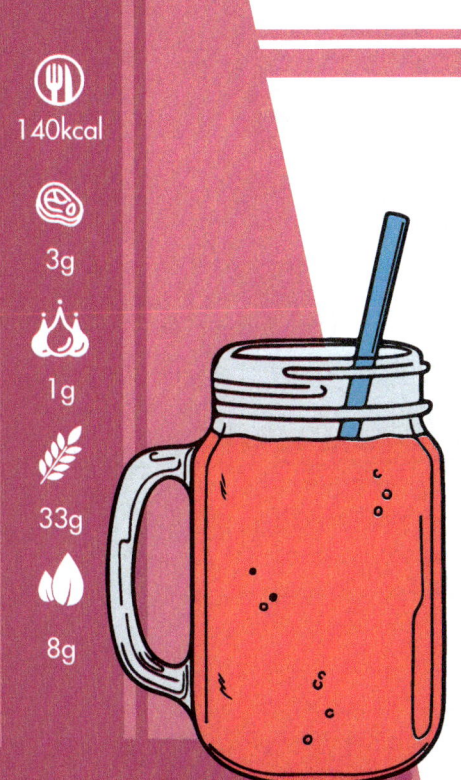

Ingredients:

- 1 cup mixed berries (strawberries, blueberries, raspberries)
- 1 small cooked beet
- 1/2 cup orange juice

Add all the ingredients to the blender and blend untill the desired texture and consistency is reached

COCONUT PINEAPPLE REFRESHER

170kcal
2g
9g
23g
2g

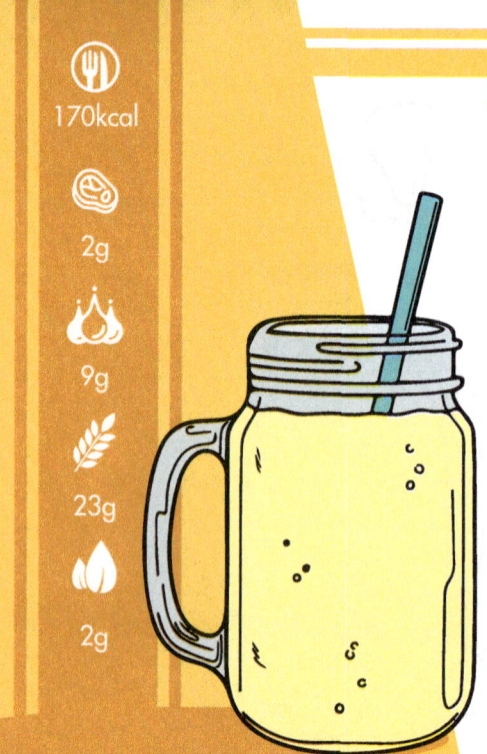

Ingredients:

- 1 cup fresh pineapple chunks
- 1/2 cup coconut water
- 1/2 cup coconut milk

Add all the ingredients to the blender and blend untill the desired texture and consistency is reached

TROPICAL SUNRISE

Ingredients:

- 1 ripe banana
- 1 cup mango chunks
- 1/2 cup orange juice

Add all the ingredients to the blender and blend untill the desired texture and consistency is reached

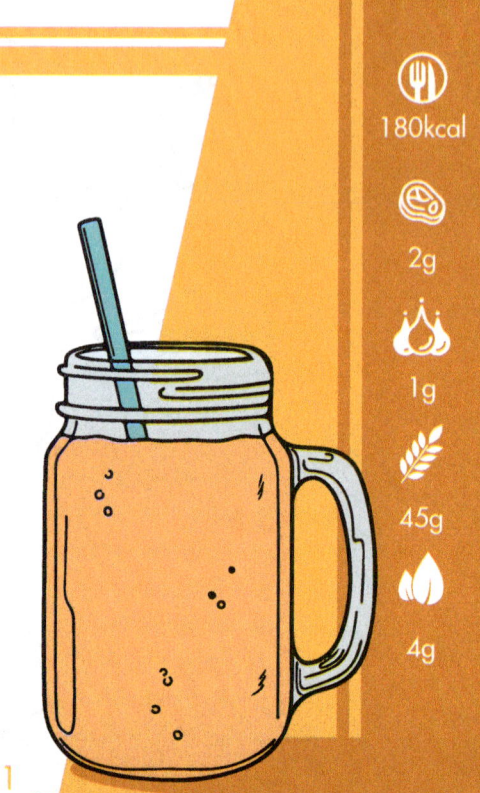

180kcal
2g
1g
45g
4g

PEANUT BUTTER BLISS

Ingredients:

- 1 ripe banana
- 1 cup almond milk
- 1 tablespoon peanut butter

Add all the ingredients to the blender and blend untill the desired texture and consistency is reached

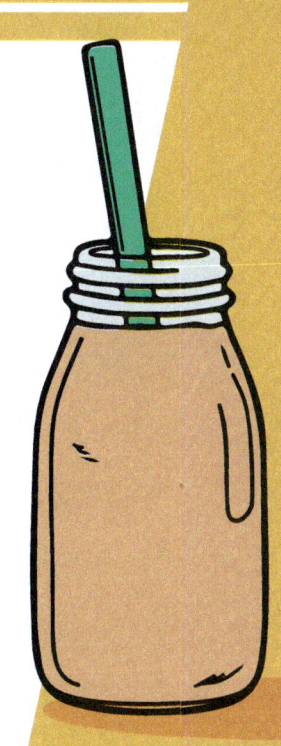

220kcal

6g

9g

32g

4g

STRAWBERRY KIWI CRUSH

Ingredients:

- 1 cup fresh strawberries
- 1 ripe kiwi
- 1/2 cup orange juice

Add all the ingredients to the blender and blend untill the desired texture and consistency is reached

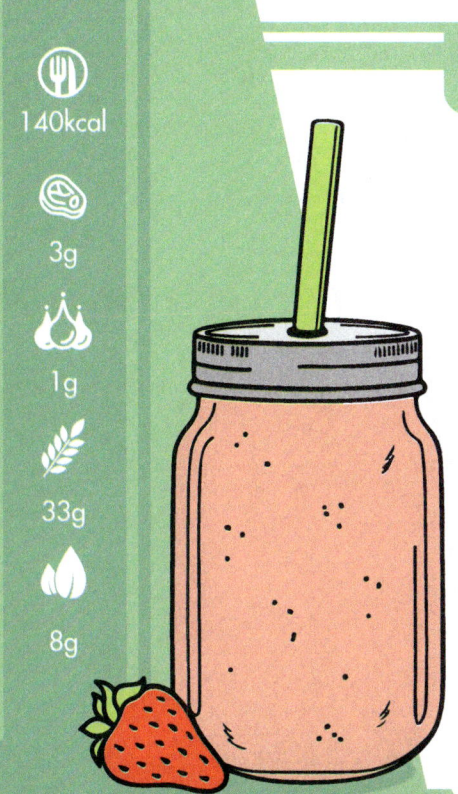

140kcal

3g

1g

33g

8g

WATERMELON LIME SPLASH

80kcal
1g
0g
20g
1g

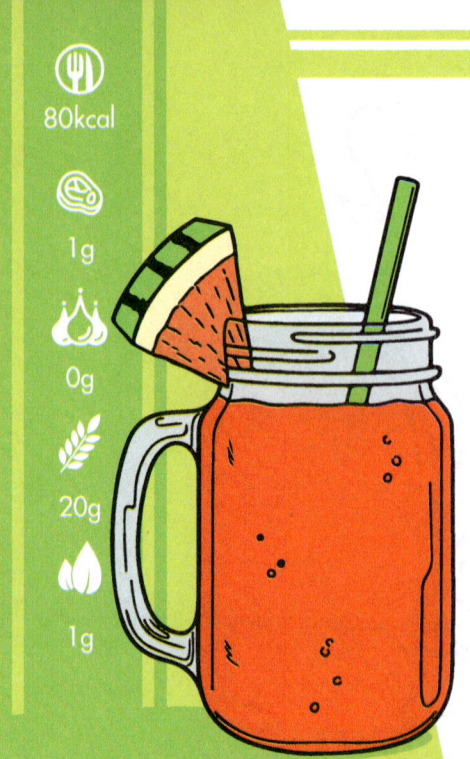

Ingredients:

- 2 cups fresh watermelon chunks
- Juice of 1 lime
- 1/2 cup coconut water

Add all the ingredients to the blender and blend untill the desired texture and consistency is reached

BLUEBERRY DELIGHT

Ingredients:

- 1 cup fresh or frozen blueberries
- 1/2 cup almond milk
- 1 tablespoon honey (optional)

Add all the ingredients to the blender and blend untill the desired texture and consistency is reached

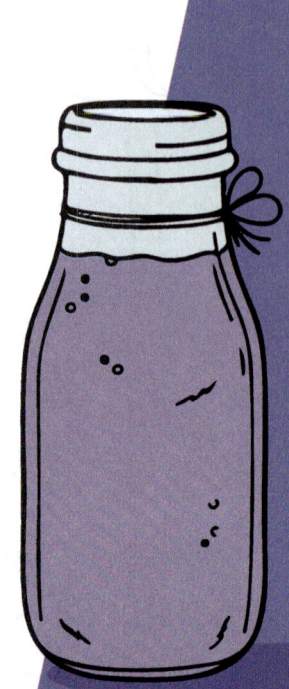

100kcal
1g
2g
24g
4g

53

CHOCOLATE BANANA SHAKE

Ingredients:

- 1 ripe banana
- 1 cup almond milk
- 1 tablespoon cocoa powder

Add all the ingredients to the blender and blend untill the desired texture and consistency is reached

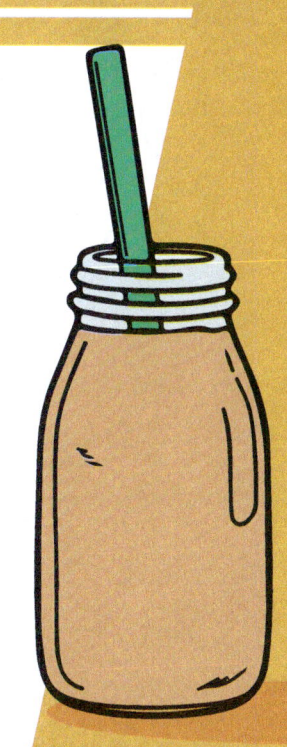

 160kcal
 4g
 4g
 32g
 6g

RASPBERRY LEMONADE

Ingredients:

- 1 cup fresh or frozen raspberries
- Juice of 1 lemon
- 1/2 cup coconut water

Add all the ingredients to the blender and blend untill the desired texture and consistency is reached

70kcal
1g
1g
18g
8g

We ran out of smoothie recipes.
Make your own.

You think you can do better than us?
Send us your creations and maybe we'll put you in the book.

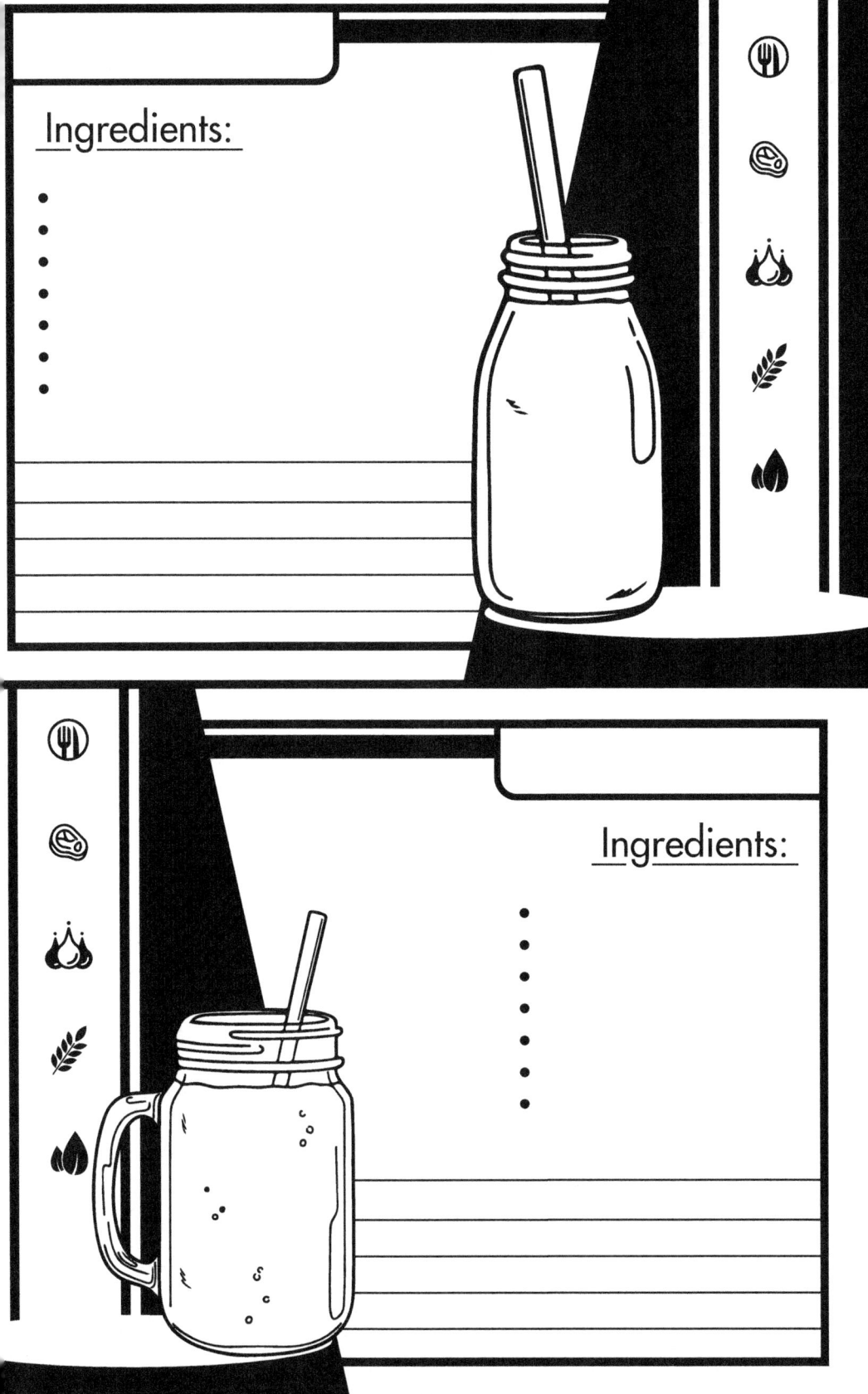

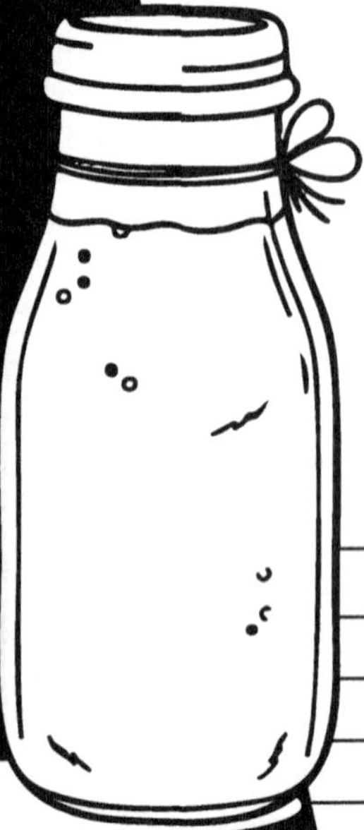

Ingredients:

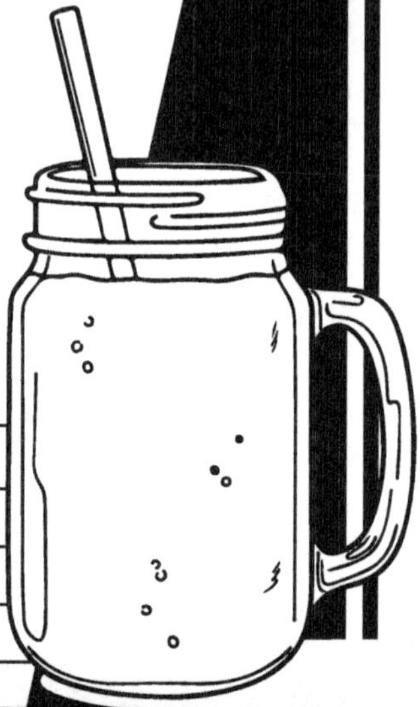

-
-
-
-
-

Ingredients:

-
-
-
-
-

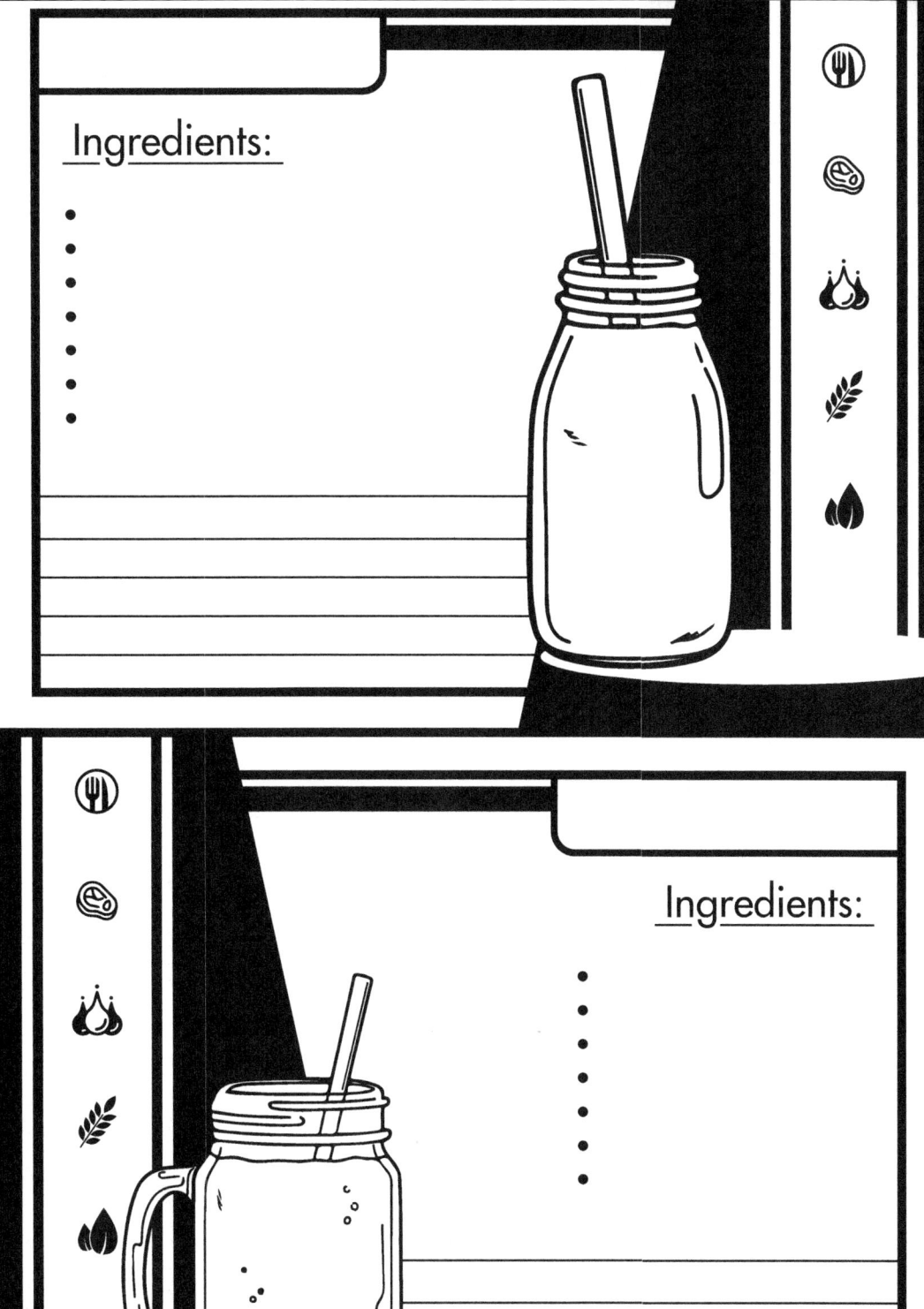

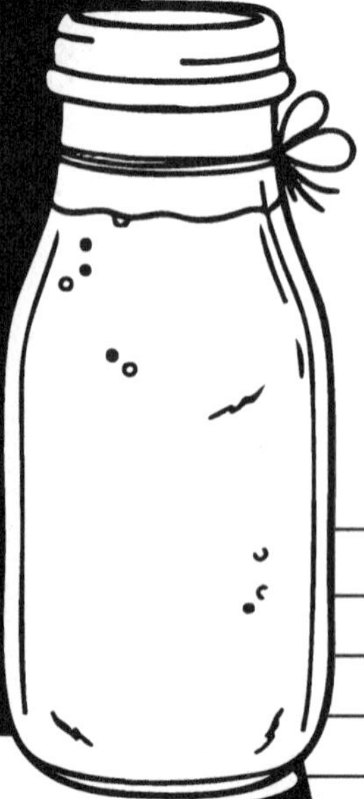

Ingredients:

-
-
-
-

Ingredients:

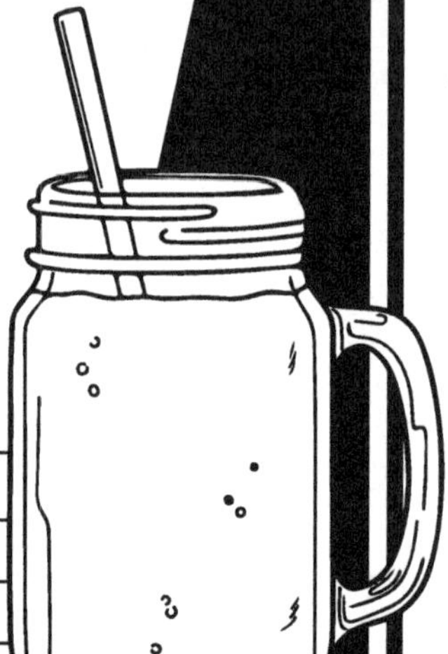

-
-
-
-
-
-

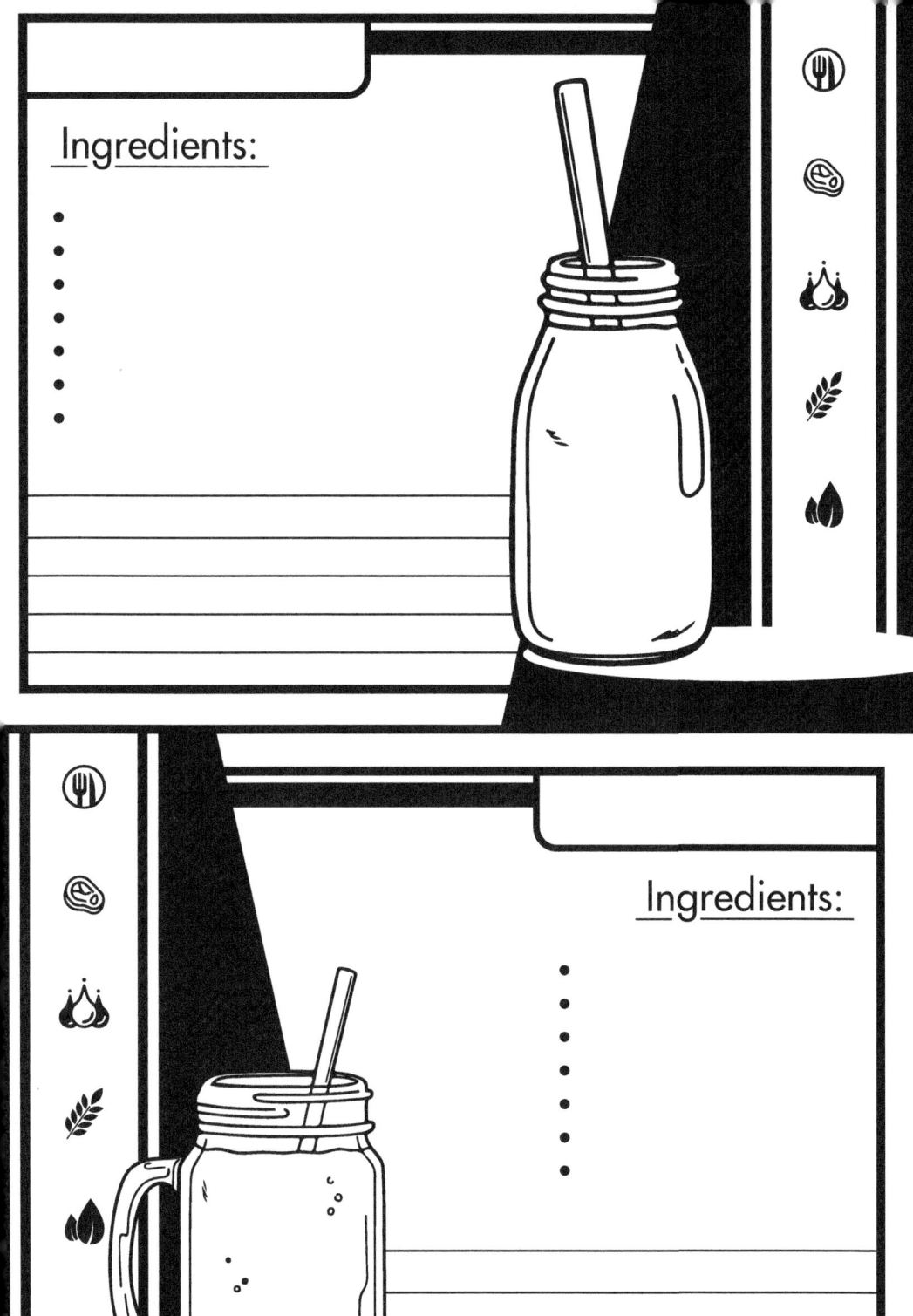

Ingredients:
-
-
-
-
-

Ingredients:
-
-
-
-
-

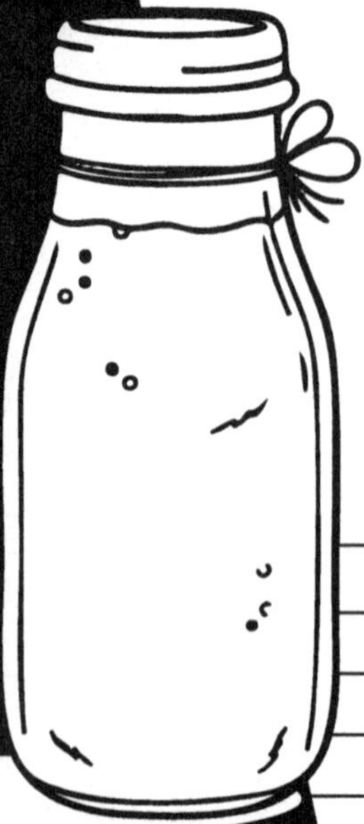

Ingredients:

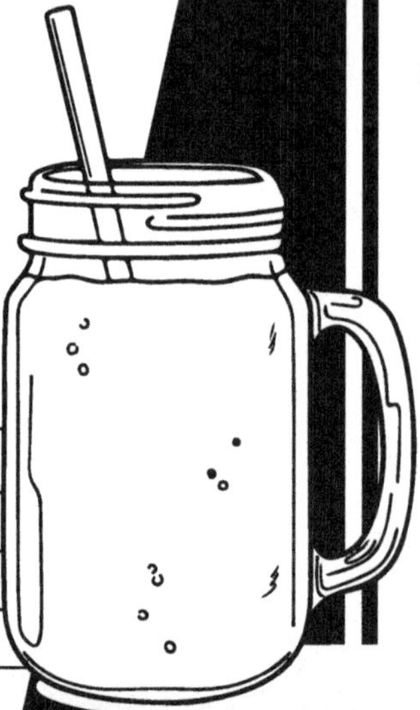

-
-
-
-
-

Ingredients:

-
-
-
-
-

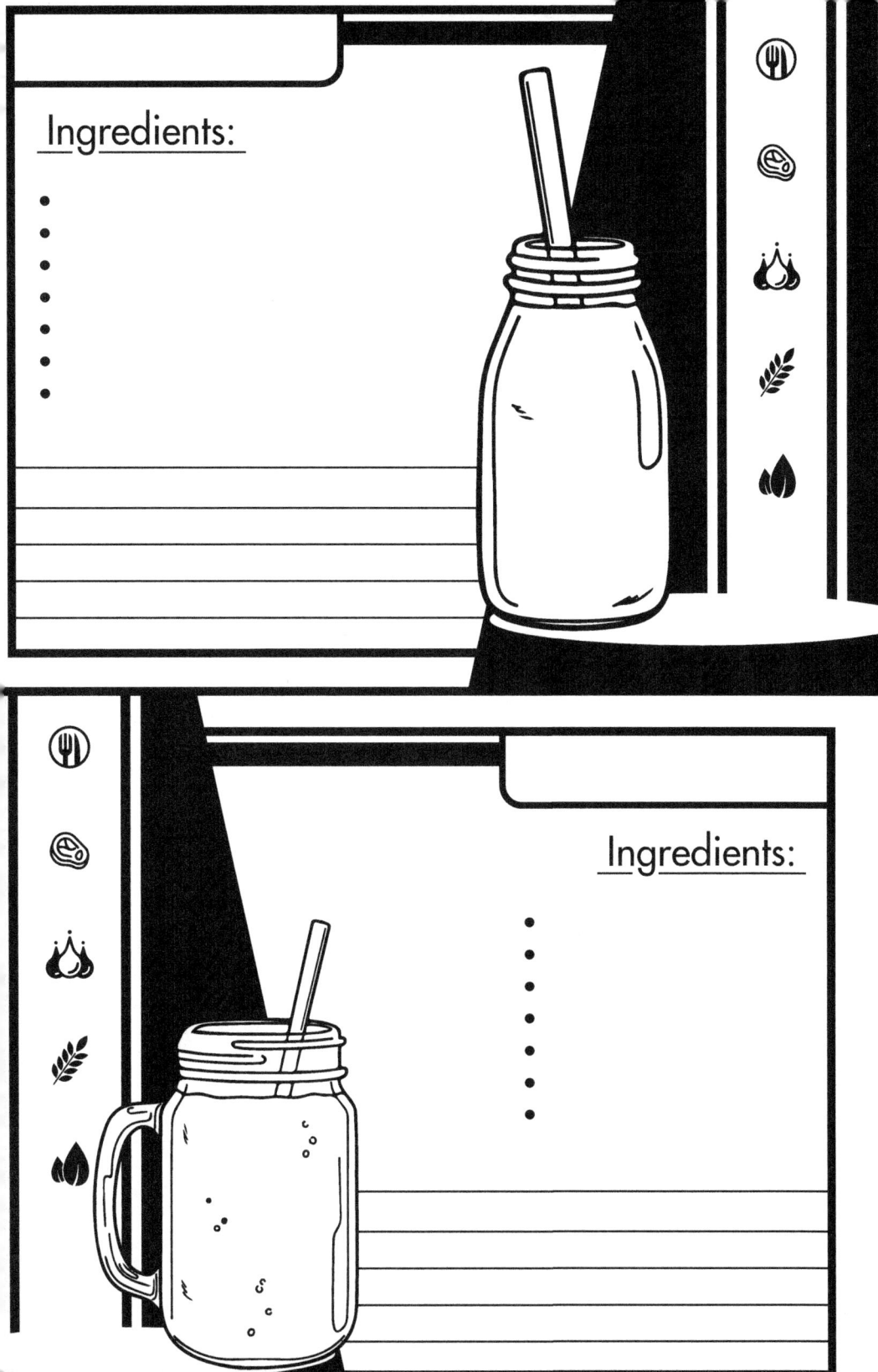

Ingredients:

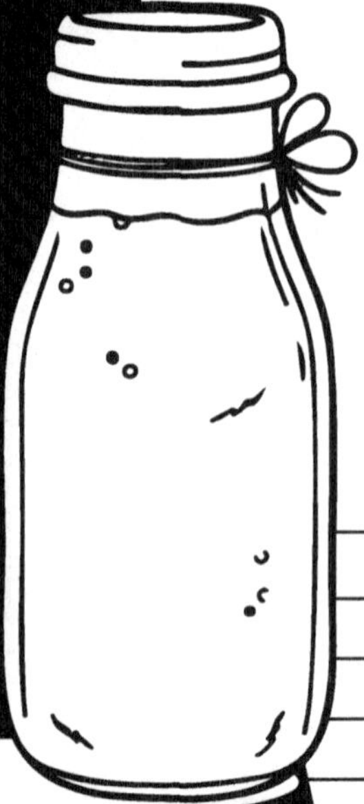

-
-
-
-
-

Ingredients:

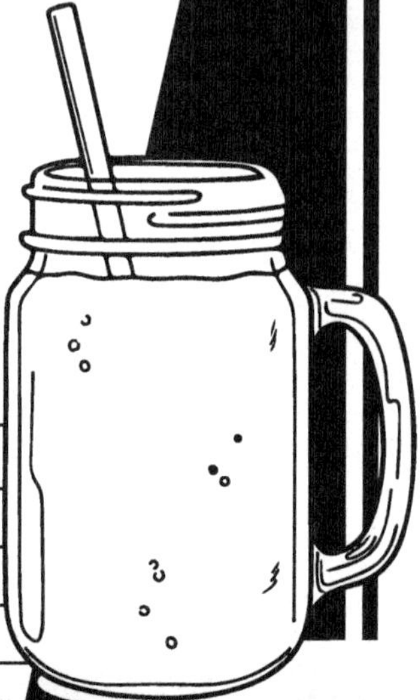

-
-
-
-
-

Ingredients:

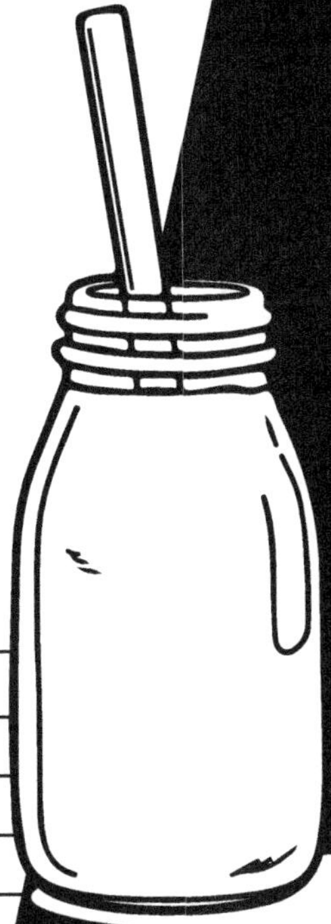

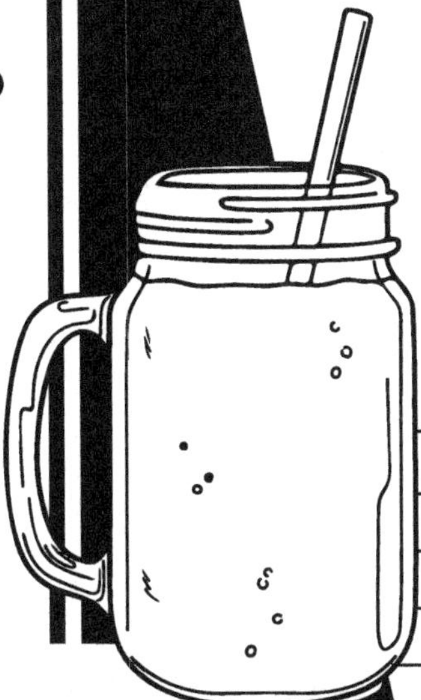

-
-
-
-
-

Ingredients:

-
-
-
-
-

INDEX

3 Ingredient Smoothies 47
A
Apple Cinnamon Detox 33
Autumn Spice 46
Avocado Detox 35
Avocado Green Dream 18
B
Banana Berry Blast 22
Banana Berry Blast 48
Banana Berry Boost 38
Banana Peanut Butter Bliss 10
Berry Beet Blend 50
Berry Detox Blast 36
Berry Oat Burst 41
Blackberry Banana Blitz 14
Blueberry Almond Delight 24
Blueberry Beet Detox 33
Blueberry Blast 6
Blueberry Delight 53
Blueberry Oat Powerhouse 29
C
Carrot Ginger Detox 34
Cherry Berry Burst 12
Chocolate Banana Power 40
Chocolate Banana Shake 54
Chocolate Cherry Powerhouse 25
Chocolate Peanut Butter Power 22
Citrus Energy Blast 40
Citrus Sunshine 10
Classic Green Goddess 16
Coconut Pineapple Refresher 51
Coffee Banana Kickstart 42
Coffee Protein Kick 26
Creamy Avocado Delight 50
Cucumber Lemon Detox 32
Cucumber Melon Cooler 17
D
Detox Smoothies 31
Disclaimer/Nutrition Symbols 3
E
Energy Smoothies 37
F
Fall Harvest 44
Fruit Smoothies 4
G
Ginger Greens 20
Ginger Turmeric Detox 34
Greek Yogurt Berry Blend 28
Green Apple Spinach Splash 20
Green Apple Zing 9
Green Goodness 49
Green Power protein Shake 29
Green Powerhouse 38
Green Protein Boost 23
Green Smoothies 15
I
Index 65
Introduction 1

Introduction 2
K
Kale Berry Blast 16
Kiwi Delight 7
L
Lemon Blueberry Refresher 13
M
Mango Berry Medley 9
Mango Ginger Zing 39
Mango Tango 48
Mango Tango 5
Matcha Green Tea Boost 42
Melon Mint Madness 14
Minty Green Refresher 19
Mixed Berry Blast 11
P
Papaya Ginger Detox 36
Peachy Keen 6
Peanut Butter Banana Boost 25
Peanut Butter Banana Boost 28
Peanut Butter Bliss 52
Pearfectly Sweet 12
Pineapple Coconut Delight 30
Pineapple Coconut Delight 39
Pineapple Kale Detox 32
Pineapple Paradise 49
Pineapple Paradise 8
Pineapple Spinach Splash 18
Protein Smoothies 21
Protein Smoothies 27
R
Raspberry Coconut Crush 13
Raspberry Lemonade 54
Raspberry Refresher 7
Raspberry Yogurt Protein 26
S
Seasonal Smoothies 43
Spinach Mango Tango 17
Spring Blossom 46
Spring Green 45
Strawberry Banana Bliss 5
Strawberry Cashew Cream 30
Strawberry Kiwi Crush 52
Summer Sunshine 44
T
Tropical Delight 11
Tropical Green Energizer 41
Tropical Green Paradise 19
Tropical Mango Protein 24
Tropical Sunrise 51
V
Vanilla Berry Protein 23
W
Watermelon Cooler 8
Watermelon Lime Splash 53
Watermelon Mint Detox 35
Winter Wonderland 45

Printed in Great Britain
by Amazon